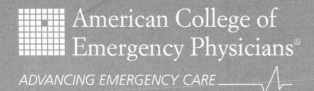
American College of
Emergency Physicians®

ADVANCING EMERGENCY CARE

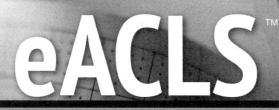
eACLS™

Advanced Cardiovascular Life Support

COURSE MANUAL

Stephen J. Rahm, NRP

Medical Editor:
Jacqueline A. Nemer, MD, FACEP

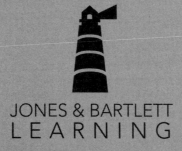

JONES & BARTLETT
LEARNING

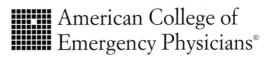

ADVANCING EMERGENCY CARE

World Headquarters
Jones & Bartlett Learning
5 Wall Street
Burlington, MA 01803
978-443-5000
info@jblearning.com
www.jblearning.com

1125 Executive Circle
Irving, TX 75038
Post Office Box 619911
Dallas, TX 75261-9911
www.acep.org

Jones & Bartlett Learning books and products are available through most bookstores and online booksellers. To contact Jones & Bartlett Learning directly, call 800-832-0034, fax 978-443-8000, or visit our website, www.jblearning.com.

Copyright © 2015 by Jones & Bartlett Learning, LLC, an Ascend Learning Company

The procedures and protocols in this book are based on the most current recommendations of responsible medical sources. ACEP and the publisher, however, make no guarantee as to, and assume no responsibility for, the correctness, sufficiency, or completeness of such information or recommendations. Other or additional safety measures may be required under particular circumstances.

This textbook is intended solely as a guide to the appropriate procedures to be employed when rendering emergency care to the sick and injured. It is not intended as a statement of the standards of care required in any particular situation, because circumstances and the patient's physical condition can vary widely from one emergency to another. Nor is it intended that this textbook shall in any way advise emergency personnel concerning legal authority to perform the activities or procedures discussed. Such local determination should be made only with the aid of legal counsel.

The American College of Emergency Physicians (ACEP) makes every effort to ensure that contributors to its publications are knowledgeable subject matter experts. Readers are nevertheless advised that the statements and opinions expressed in this publication are provided as the contributors' recommendations at the time of publication and should not be construed as official College policy. ACEP recognizes the complexity of emergency medicine and makes no representation that this publication serves as an authoritative resource for the prevention, diagnosis, treatment, or intervention for any medical condition, nor should it be the basis for definition of, or standard of care that should be practiced by all health care providers at any particular time or place. To the fullest extent permitted by law, and without limitation, ACEP expressly disclaims all liability for errors or omissions contained within this publication, and for damages of any kind or nature, arising out of use, reference to, reliance on, or performance of such information.

Production Credits
Chief Executive Officer: Ty Field
President: James Homer
EVP, Chief Product Officer: Ed Moura
Executive Publisher: Kimberly Brophy
Executive Acquisitions Editor—EMS: Christine Emerton
Managing Editor: Carol B. Guerrero
Senior Editor: Jennifer Deforge-Kling
Associate Director, Production: Jenny Corriveau

Director of Marketing: Alisha Weisman
V.P., Manufacturing and Inventory Control: Therese Connell
Composition: Cenveo Publisher Services
Cover Design: Michael O'Donnell
Director, Permissions and Photo Research: Amy Wrynn
Cover Image: © Comstock/Thinkstock
Printing and Binding: Courier Companies
Cover Printing: Courier Companies

Library of Congress Cataloging-in-Publication Data
Rahm, Stephen J.
   eACLS : advanced cardiovascular life support course manual / Stephen J. Rahm. 3rd ed.
      p. ; cm.
   Includes index.
   Rev. ed. of: eACLS study guide. 2nd ed. 2007.
   ISBN 978-1-4496-4185-6
   I. Rahm, Stephen J. eACLS study guide. II. American College of Emergency Physicians. III. Title.
   [DNLM: 1. Advanced Cardiac Life Support. WG 205]

   616.1'2025—dc23
                  2012037096
6048

Printed in the United States of America
18 17 16 15 14   10 9 8 7 6 5 4 3 2 1

CONTENTS

Chapter 2: Pharmacologic and Electrical Therapy 15

Chapter 3: Patient Assessment and eACLS Case Review 27

Chapter 4: eACLS Practice Cases 53

Appendix A: eACLS Practice Test............ 72

Introduction

Welcome to eACLS™! The "e" refers to electronic, efficient, and easy. ACLS refers to Advanced Cardiovascular Life Support. This course manual has been developed to assist you, the ACLS provider or instructor, in reviewing the principles and concepts of managing a patient with a respiratory or cardiovascular system emergency. This information and activities in this course manual are intended to accommodate both those who are relatively new to ACLS and the experienced provider.

The eACLS™ course and this course manual provide you with the opportunity to review your baseline knowledge of the following key components of advanced cardiovascular care:

- Cardiac rhythms

- Pharmacologic therapy

- Electrical therapy

- Patient assessment

Specific practice cases are presented in this course manual and the eACLS™ course that incorporate the above key components. These cases include:

- Acute coronary syndromes (ACS)
- Asystole
- Bradycardia
- Pulseless electrical activity
- Stroke
- Tachycardia – narrow complex
- Tachycardia – wide complex
- Ventricular fibrillation

Each case will present a patient, the patient's chief complaint, the ECG tracing if applicable, and the initial examination findings. After being provided with this information, you must decide which treatment algorithm/approach would be most appropriate for the patient.

Within each case, you will be asked questions about the assessment and treatment that you would provide for the patient. More challenging questions will be identified as **"Beyond eACLS Basics."** A summary, which contains the answers and rationales for the practice case questions, will immediately follow each practice case.

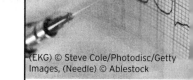
At the end of this course manual, you will find a comprehensive practice written examination, which has 40 randomly developed items from all of the eACLS™ core cases. The answers, along with rationales for both correct and incorrect responses, will immediately follow the practice written examination.

The eACLS™ Course

eACLS™ is a highly interactive program that allows healthcare professionals to show their competency, as well as earn national certification, as an ACLS provider.

Each of the eACLS™ case studies has the following components:

- Case introduction known as "Your Patient," which covers your initial patient presentation

- Assessment tutorial

- Treatment tutorial

- Interactivities with multiple-choice, fill-in-the-blank, and matching exercises that assess your understanding of the key concepts for each case

- A highly interactive simulation, which puts you in the driver's seat of assessing and managing the patient

You must successfully complete all of these components in each case before you will be able to move on to another case.

The final written exam is composed of 40 multiple-choice, case-based questions (5 per case study). The questions are based on the objectives of the case studies and include ECGs when appropriate. Each question is worth 2.5 points. Once the exam is completed, it is graded instantly. You must score at least 80% to pass the course. If you fail the first exam, you will have an opportunity to remediate by viewing the eACLS™ course cases and Resources Section, before attempting the exam again. If you fail the second exam, remediation is offered on all questions and you will be advised to retake the eACLS™ course.

Feel free to use this course manual as a preparatory tool for eACLS™ as well as a reference tool during the program itself. We are confident that you will find eACLS™ to be an interactive experience that is both engaging and educational.

Review of Cardiac Rhythms

Introduction

This chapter focuses primarily on the cardiac rhythms addressed in eACLS and is not intended to be inclusive of all cardiac rhythms that may be encountered by the health care provider. Clinicians are encouraged to refer to the text *Arrhythmia Recognition: The Art of Interpretation* by Tomas B. Garcia, MD, and Geoffrey T. Miller, NREMT-P (Jones & Bartlett Publishers, 2004) for a detailed review of the cardiac electrical conduction system, including all cardiac rhythm disturbances and their variants.

It is important to identify the specific cardiac rhythm disturbance presenting on the electrocardiogram (ECG). It is equally, if not more, important to recognize whether the patient is hemodynamically stable or unstable as a result of the cardiac rhythm disturbance. This status determines the most appropriate treatment approach.

Cardiac Electrical Conduction System

Conduction System Components

As you will recall, the myocardium is a unique muscle in the human body. It has the ability to generate its own electricity, a process called automacity. A pacemaker is a collection of myocardial cells that set the inherent rate of electrical discharge for the heart. Electrical impulses are generated by a pacemaker and then transmitted in an organized fashion, throughout the myocardium by way of a specialized conduction system (**FIGURE 1-1**).

In a normal heart, the primary pacemaker is the sinoatrial (SA) node, also referred to as the sinus node. The SA node is located in the superior aspect of the right atrium and inherently discharges 60–100 electrical impulses per minute in adults.

Once initiated in the SA node, the electrical impulse travels, via the internodal pathways, throughout the right and left atria and depolarizes their cells. This depolarization (electrical discharge) stimulates the atrial muscle to contract.

The impulse travels farther to the atrioventricular (AV) node, where it is delayed briefly before entering the ventricles. This delay is necessary to allow the ventricles to fill completely prior to the onset of ventricular contraction. The AV node is located at the base of the right atrium in the center of the heart where all four chambers come together.

If for some reason the SA node fails as the primary pacemaker, the AV node can assume the responsibility of pacing the heart. However, it does so at a slower rate, with an inherent discharge rate of 40–60 electrical impulses per minute. After the brief AV nodal delay, the

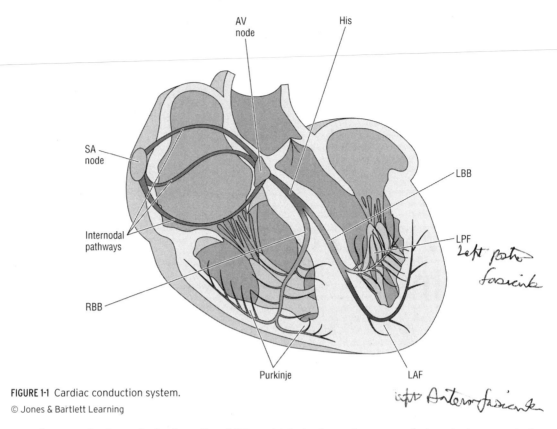

FIGURE 1-1 Cardiac conduction system.

© Jones & Bartlett Learning

Left posto fasciule

left Anterio fasciule

impulse travels through the bundle of His, which is the only route of electrical transmission between the atria and the ventricles.

The bundle of His, which is located partially in the walls of the right atrium and in the interventricular septum, gives rise to a right and left bundle branch, the left of which has an anterior and a posterior fascicle. The left bundle branch has two fascicles because the left ventricle is much larger than the right ventricle. The bundle branches terminate into the Purkinje system, which depolarizes the ventricular cells, thus causing the ventricular muscle to contract.

If both the SA and the AV nodes fail to generate an electrical impulse, the ventricles can become the primary pacemaker; however, they generate electricity much slower, at a rate of only 20–40 electrical impulses per minute.

ECG Waveform Representations

Each event in the cardiac conduction system produces a specific waveform that can be analyzed with an ECG. One entire cardiac cycle produces a single complex of waveforms (**FIGURE 1-2**). It is important to remember that the ECG is not a representation of myocardial mechanics; it merely

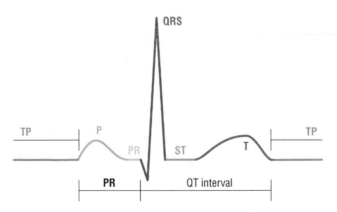

FIGURE 1-2 ECG complex waveforms.

© Jones & Bartlett Learning

depicts the electrical events that stimulate myocardial contraction. A rhythm on the ECG is not equivalent to a palpable pulse.

The P wave, which is normally upright in most leads, is the first waveform on the ECG. It represents simultaneous depolarization of both atria. The P-R segment, which is the timeframe between the end of the P wave and the beginning of the QRS complex, represents the delay at the AV node. The P-R interval, which begins at the initiation of the P wave and ends at the QRS complex, represents the entire atrial depolarization process, including the delay at the AV node.

Collectively, the QRS complex represents ventricular depolarization. The Q wave, which is the first negative deflection after the P wave, can be present or absent. Q-wave significance is discussed in the next section of this chapter. The R wave is the first positive deflection after the P wave. The S wave is the first negative deflection after the R wave.

The ST segment represents the timeframe between ventricular depolarization and repolarization. The ST segment should be isoelectric, which is the baseline of the cardiac cycle or electrically neutral. ST-segment depression or elevation of less than 1 mm may be insignificant; however, this is not conclusive. ST-segment depression and elevation are discussed in the next section of this chapter.

The T wave, which represents ventricular repolarization, is the first deflection that occurs after the ST segment. The T-wave deflection should be in the same general direction as the QRS complex. T-wave inversion is also discussed in the next section of this chapter.

Normal Sinus Rhythm (NSR)

Now that we have reviewed the cardiac electrical system and the ECG waveforms, let's look at a normal sinus rhythm. In order to recognize the abnormal, we must first recognize and appreciate the normal. A normal sinus rhythm (FIGURE 1-3) indicates that all components of the cardiac electrical system are intact and are functioning normally. Remember, it does not signify if the patient is stable or even has a pulse.

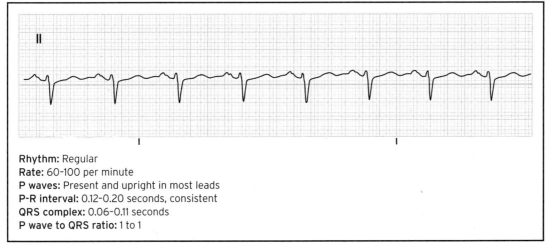

Rhythm: Regular
Rate: 60-100 per minute
P waves: Present and upright in most leads
P-R interval: 0.12-0.20 seconds, consistent
QRS complex: 0.06-0.11 seconds
P wave to QRS ratio: 1 to 1

FIGURE 1-3 Normal sinus rhythm.
From *Arrhythmia Recognition: The Art of Interpretation*, courtesy of Tomas B. Garcia, MD.

Origin

Normal sinus rhythm indicates that the SA node is the primary pacemaker site and that all components of the cardiovascular electrical system are intact and functioning normally.

Clinical Significance

There is no clinical significance, unless the normal sinus rhythm occurs in the absence of a pulse.

ECG Markers of Acute Coronary Syndrome

ST-Segment Depression and Elevation

The ST segment represents the timeframe between ventricular depolarization and repolarization. The ST segment should be at the isoelectric line (baseline), which represents the period of time when the myocardium is electrically neutral.

Slight depression and elevation (ie, <1 mm) of the ST segment in various lead configurations may be benign. Any ST-segment depression or elevation in a patient with chest pain or other signs and symptoms of an acute coronary syndrome might be significant and could represent acute myocardial ischemia or infarction until proved otherwise (FIGURE 1-4).

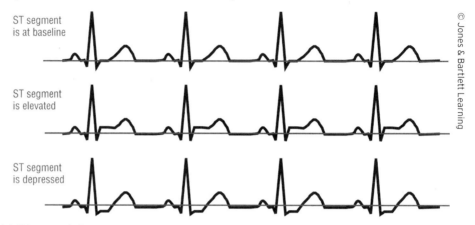

© Jones & Bartlett Learning

FIGURE 1-4 ST-segment changes.

As a general rule, ST-segment depression can occur with myocardial ischemia, and ST-segment elevation can indicate myocardial injury. The significance depends on the pattern of the ST-segment abnormality, and the presence of other causes of ST-segment deviation such as bundle branch block or hypertrophy. For these findings to be conclusive, one would need a 12-lead ECG tracing. ST segment changes cannot be assessed using a standard cardiac monitor. Cardiac monitoring shows only one lead and is not of "diagnostic quality" because electronic filtration is used to make P-waves more prominent to aid in rhythm interpretation. This filtering can distort the ST segment, causing fictitious ST-segment elevation or depression.

A 12-lead ECG is needed to aid in the diagnosis of myocardial ischemia or infarction. Although 12-lead electrocardiography is beyond the scope of this text, we must remember that a patient with an acute coronary syndrome can have a normal 12-lead ECG. This reminds us of the important concept of "treating the patient, not the monitor."

T-Wave Inversion

The T wave represents repolarization of the ventricles. Its deflection should be in the same direction as the QRS complex. An inverted T wave (FIGURE 1-5) can indicate myocardial ischemia.

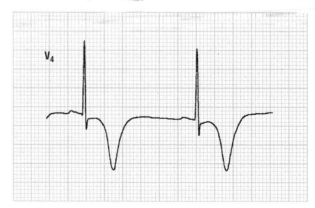

FIGURE 1-5 T-wave inversion.

Adapted from *12-Lead ECG: The Art of Interpretation*, courtesy of Tomas B. Garcia, MD.

Again, for this finding to be conclusive, a 12-lead ECG would be required for the T waves to be viewed in other leads.

Q Waves

The Q wave, if visible, is the first negative deflection after the P wave. Q waves can be clinically insignificant in some leads. A significant or "pathologic" Q wave is defined as one that is either one-third the total height of the QRS complex (FIGURE 1-6), or more than 0.03 seconds wide (FIGURE 1-7).

Pathological Q waves represent dead myocardium and indicate the occurrence and location of a previous myocardial infarction. Without the benefit of a previous 12-lead ECG tracing, one cannot conclude the age of the infarct.

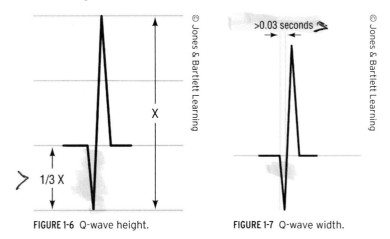

FIGURE 1-6 Q-wave height.   FIGURE 1-7 Q-wave width.

Bradycardias

Introduction

Bradycardia is defined by a heart rate of less than 60 beats per minute. This may result in a decrease in cardiac output, which may lead to a patient becoming clinically unstable if the patient's heart cannot compensate for the decreased rate by increasing its ability to pump more blood with each heartbeat. Absolute bradycardia refers to any heart rate less than 60 beats per minute (FIGURE 1-8). Relative bradycardia is a term used to describe a heart rate that is greater than 60 beats per minute but too slow given the patient's condition. For example, the patient may have a heart rate of 70 beats per minute; however, while experiencing altered mental status, hypotension, or other signs of hemodynamic compromise, this would be considered a clinically significant bradycardia because the heart rate is not adequate for the clinical situation.

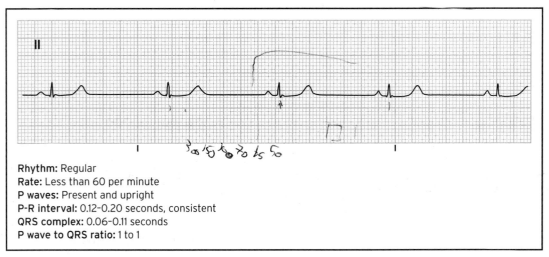

Rhythm: Regular
Rate: Less than 60 per minute
P waves: Present and upright
P-R interval: 0.12–0.20 seconds, consistent
QRS complex: 0.06–0.11 seconds
P wave to QRS ratio: 1 to 1

FIGURE 1-8 Sinus bradycardia.
From *Arrhythmia Recognition: The Art of Interpretation*, courtesy of Tomas B. Garcia, MD.

Hypoxemia is a common cause of bradycardia. Other causes of bradycardia include medications, structural damage, and metabolic dysfunction (ie, electrolytes abnormalities, thyroid disease). The ACLS algorithm is a guideline for treatment of clinically significant bradycardia.

Sinus Bradycardia

Origin

Sinus bradycardia can result from excess vagal stimulation, which slows SA node discharge. This may result from hypoxemia disease, damage to the cardiac electrical conduction system, medications, (ie, beta blockers, calcium channel blockers) and metabolic dysfunction.

Clinical Significance

Sinus bradycardia can result in a decreased cardiac output. In those who routinely engage in aerobic exercise, sinus bradycardia may be a normal finding.

Idioventricular Rhythm

Origin

Idioventricular rhythms (FIGURE 1-9) occur when a ventricular focus acts as the primary pacemaker for the heart. This is identified by a slow ventricular rate of 20–40 beats per minute and a wide and bizarre appearance of the QRS complexes. Because atrial activity is absent, there are no P waves preceding each QRS complex.

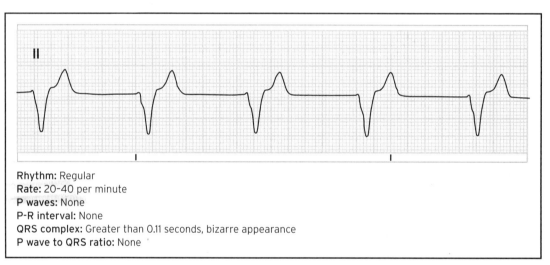

Rhythm: Regular
Rate: 20-40 per minute
P waves: None
P-R interval: None
QRS complex: Greater than 0.11 seconds, bizarre appearance
P wave to QRS ratio: None

FIGURE 1-9 Idioventricular rhythm.

From *Arrhythmia Recognition: The Art of Interpretation*, courtesy of Tomas B. Garcia, MD.

Clinical Significance

This idioventricular rhythm may result in decreased cardiac output and poor perfusion. In the absence of atrial contraction, a reduced volume of blood is ejected into the ventricles. Additionally, the ventricular rate is slow, which may result in a reduced cardiac output.

Heart Blocks

Atrioventricular (AV) heart blocks are caused by the electrical conduction through the AV node. These are classified as first degree, second degree (Mobitz type I and II), and third degree.

Origin: First-Degree Heart Block

First-degree AV block (FIGURE 1-10) is a prolonged P-R interval beyond 0.20 seconds. Factors such as vagal stimulation, AV nodal disease, and certain medications can cause this cardiac rhythm.

Clinical Significance

When first-degree AV block is associated with bradycardia, cardiac output can fall. First-degree AV block may be a normal variant in some people. This is typically a benign rhythm.

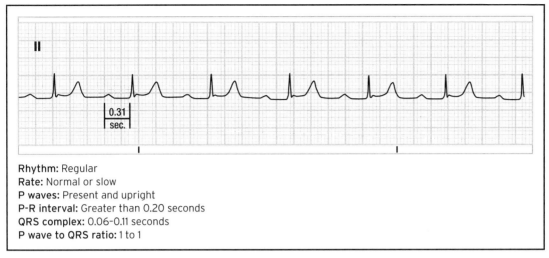

Rhythm: Regular
Rate: Normal or slow
P waves: Present and upright
P-R interval: Greater than 0.20 seconds
QRS complex: 0.06-0.11 seconds
P wave to QRS ratio: 1 to 1

FIGURE 1-10 First-degree AV block.

From *Arrhythmia Recognition: The Art of Interpretation*, courtesy of Tomas B. Garcia, MD.

Origin: Second-Degree Heart Block—Mobitz Type I

Second-degree AV Mobitz type I block is at the AV node (FIGURE 1-11). Each atrial conducted complex has a progressive widening of the P-R interval, followed by a QRS complex that is progressively delayed at the AV node until it is completely blocked, which results in a "stand alone" P wave that is not followed by a QRS complex. Mobitz type 1 block is commonly transient and caused by AV nodal disease, medications, and vagal stimulation.

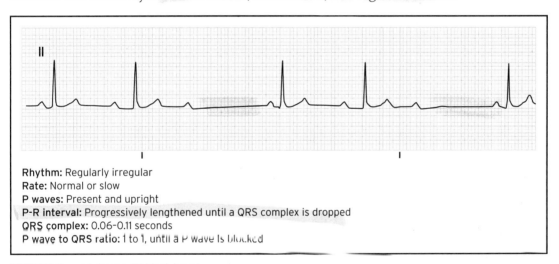

Rhythm: Regularly irregular
Rate: Normal or slow
P waves: Present and upright
P-R interval: Progressively lengthened until a QRS complex is dropped
QRS complex: 0.06-0.11 seconds
P wave to QRS ratio: 1 to 1, until a P wave is blocked

FIGURE 1-11 Second-degree AV block type I.

From *Arrhythmia Recognition: The Art of Interpretation*, courtesy of Tomas B. Garcia, MD.

Clinical Significance

This cardiac rhythm can either present with a normal or a bradycardic rate. If second-degree AV block type I is associated with bradycardia, cardiac output may decrease.

Origin: Second-Degree Heart Block—Mobitz Type II

Second-degree AV block Mobitz type II (FIGURE 1-12) usually occurs when the block is below the AV node. Some atrial conducted complexes are blocked by the AV node intermittently. This results in some P waves that are not followed by a QRS complex.

Clinical Significance

Second-degree AV block type II usually results from more severe AV nodal disease below the bundle of His. Because of this, Mobitz type II block is frequently symptomatic and may deteriorate suddenly into a third-degree block.

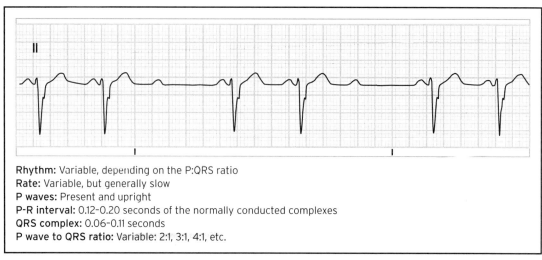

Rhythm: Variable, depending on the P:QRS ratio
Rate: Variable, but generally slow
P waves: Present and upright
P-R interval: 0.12-0.20 seconds of the normally conducted complexes
QRS complex: 0.06-0.11 seconds
P wave to QRS ratio: Variable: 2:1, 3:1, 4:1, etc.

FIGURE 1-12 Second-degree AV block type II.
From *Arrhythmia Recognition: The Art of Interpretation*, courtesy of Tomas B. Garcia, MD.

Origin: Third-Degree Heart Block

Third-degree complete AV block (**FIGURE 1-13**) occurs when electrical conduction is completely blocked between atria and ventricles. This block may be located within the AV node, bundle of His, or bundle branches. As a result, the ventricles respond with escape complexes, thus producing a wide QRS complex.

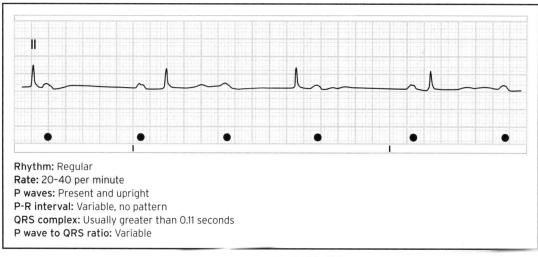

Rhythm: Regular
Rate: 20-40 per minute
P waves: Present and upright
P-R interval: Variable, no pattern
QRS complex: Usually greater than 0.11 seconds
P wave to QRS ratio: Variable

FIGURE 1-13 Third-degree AV block
From *Arrhythmia Recognition: The Art of Interpretation*, courtesy of Tomas B. Garcia, MD.

Clinical Significance

When atrial and ventricular contractions are dissociated, cardiac output may decrease and the patient may become clinically unstable. Because the atrial conducted complexes are blocked at the AV node, a ventricular pacemaker initiates an impulse at its inherent rate of 20–40 beats per minute, which produces wide QRS complexes. Third-degree block may be transient or permanent, depending upon the circumstance.

Tachycardias

Introduction

Tachycardia is defined as a heart rate that is greater than 100 beats per minute in adults. Tachycardia is categorized based on heart rate, regularity, and morphology of QRS complex (<0.12 second) vs wide (0.12 second or greater). If the heart beats too fast, the ventricles may not fill adequately. This could result in a decrease in cardiac output, poor perfusion, and hemodynamic instability. ACLS guidelines use the terms "narrow complex" and "wide complex" instead of supraventricular (SVT) and ventricular tachycardia (V-tach) because it can be difficult to identify whether a rhythm is supraventricular or ventricular in origin. Tachycardia is often due to hypoxemia, medications, structural damage, and metabolic dysfunction (ie, electrolytes abnormalities, thyroid disease). Tachycardia requires treatment if there is rate-related hemodynamic instability (ie, altered mental status, hypotension, cardiac ischemia).

Narrow QRS Complex
Origin: Sinus Tachycardia

Sinus tachycardia (**FIGURE 1-14**) occurs when the SA node discharges faster than its inherent rate of 60–100 electrical impulses per minute. This can be caused by certain medications or by situations (ie, shock, fever, hypoxemia, exercise).

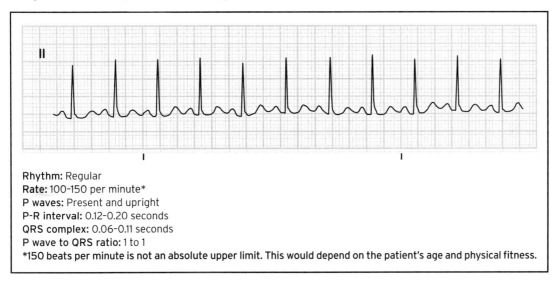

Rhythm: Regular
Rate: 100-150 per minute*
P waves: Present and upright
P-R interval: 0.12-0.20 seconds
QRS complex: 0.06-0.11 seconds
P wave to QRS ratio: 1 to 1
*150 beats per minute is not an absolute upper limit. This would depend on the patient's age and physical fitness.

FIGURE 1-14 Sinus tachycardia.

From *Arrhythmia Recognition: The Art of Interpretation*, courtesy of Tomas B. Garcia, MD.

Clinical Significance

Sinus tachycardia rarely results in a decreased cardiac output secondary to inadequate ventricular filling. More commonly sinus tachycardia preserves cardiac output by acting to compensate for other conditions (ie, moderate blood loss).

Narrow complex tachycardia is also commonly referred to as supraventricular tachycardia (SVT) (**FIGURE 1-15**). SVTs include many rhythms listed in order of frequency: atrial fibrillation and flutter, AV nodal reentry, accessory pathway-mediated, atrial, multifocal, and junctional tachycardia. For the purposes of this review, we define SVT as being a narrow-complex

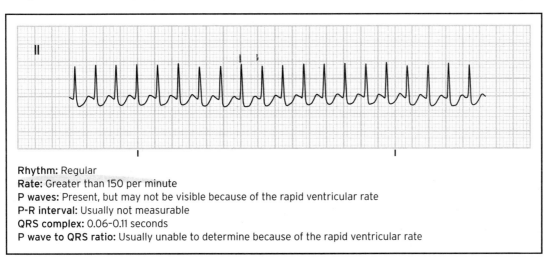

Rhythm: Regular
Rate: Greater than 150 per minute
P waves: Present, but may not be visible because of the rapid ventricular rate
P-R interval: Usually not measurable
QRS complex: 0.06-0.11 seconds
P wave to QRS ratio: Usually unable to determine because of the rapid ventricular rate

FIGURE 1-15 Supraventricular tachycardia (SVT).

From *Arrhythmia Recognition: The Art of Interpretation*, courtesy of Tomas B. Garcia, MD.

tachycardia with a heart rate that exceeds 150 beats per minute that typically starts and stops suddenly, as opposed to sinus tachycardia, which usually speeds up and slows down gradually.

Origin: Paroxysmal Supraventricular Tachycardia

Paroxysmal supraventricular tachycardia (PSVT) occurs when a supraventricular (above the ventricles) pacemaker other than the SA node initiates the cardiac cycle. PSVT is the original and commonly used term to describe reentry tachycardias. It is important to distinguish between the reentry SVTs which are located in the atria (ie, atrial fibrillation and flutter) and those that involve the AV node since this determines treatment response. Like sinus tachycardia, PSVT can be caused by certain medications or situations (ie, shock, fever, hypoxemia, exercise) as well as disease of the SA node or a reentry circuit in the AV node.

Clinical Significance

PSVT with a very fast ventricular rate can result in inadequate ventricular filling, decreased cardiac output, and poor perfusion.

Origin: Atrial Fibrillation

Atrial fibrillation (**FIGURE 1-16**) is the result of multiple atrial pacemakers discharging chaotically. As a result, there are no discernible P waves, but rather fibrillatory waves between each QRS complex. Because there is no coordinated electrical pattern from the atria to the ventricles, electricity traverses the AV node sporadically, resulting in a ventricular rhythm that is irregularly irregular.

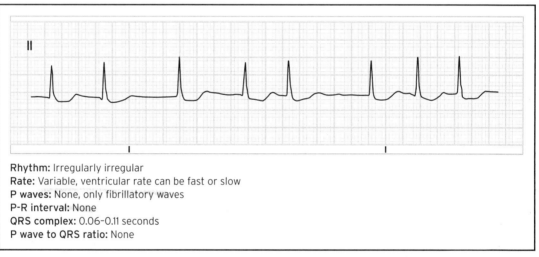

Rhythm: Irregularly irregular
Rate: Variable, ventricular rate can be fast or slow
P waves: None, only fibrillatory waves
P-R interval: None
QRS complex: 0.06-0.11 seconds
P wave to QRS ratio: None

FIGURE 1-16 Atrial fibrillation.

From *Arrhythmia Recognition: The Art of Interpretation*, courtesy of Tomas B. Garcia, MD.

Clinical Significance

Atrial fibrillation is frequently encountered in patients with congestive heart failure or SA node damage, or conduction system dysfunction from damage, disease, drugs, or metabolic disorders. Several potential problems are associated with this dysrhythmia. First, because the atria are fibrillating, blood has a tendency to stagnate, which increases the risk of microemboli formation and subsequent pulmonary, coronary, or cerebral embolism. Second, when the ventricular rate of atrial fibrillation exceeds 100 beats per minute, cardiac output can decrease. This decrease in cardiac output is compounded by the loss of atrial kick because smaller volumes of blood are ejected into the ventricles from the fibrillating atria.

Origin: Atrial Flutter

Atrial flutter (**FIGURE 1-17**) is the result of an ectopic atrial pacemaker or the site of a rapid reentry circuit within the atria, but outside of the SA node. The ectopic pacemaker is commonly in the lower atrium, near the AV node. SA node function is completely suppressed by atrial flutter. Instead of P waves, atrial flutter produces flutter (F) waves, as a result of the depolarization of the atria in an abnormal manner. The classic F waves of atrial flutter resemble a sawtooth.

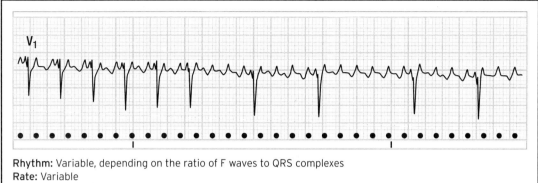

Rhythm: Variable, depending on the ratio of F waves to QRS complexes
Rate: Variable
P waves: Sawtooth appearance, flutter (F) waves
P-R interval: Variable
QRS complex: 0.06-0.11 seconds
P wave to QRS ratio: F wave to QRS ratio is variable, but most commonly 2:1

FIGURE 1-17 Atrial flutter.

From *Arrhythmia Recognition: The Art of Interpretation*, courtesy of Tomas B. Garcia, MD.

Clinical Significance

Atrial flutter usually occurs in patients with underlying structural heart disease. As with atrial fibrillation, complications occur with this dysrhythmia as a result of inadequate ventricular filling, especially when it is accompanied by a rapid ventricular rate. Cardiac output can decrease significantly if there is a very fast ventricular response rate.

Wide QRS Complex

Origin: Monomorphic Ventricular Tachycardia

Most wide complex tachycardias (WCT) originate in a ventricle. Common WCTs include: ventricular tachycardia, ventricular fibrillation, SVT with aberrancy, pre-excited tachycardias, and ventricular paced rhythms. The most common form is monomorphic ventricular tachycardia (FIGURE 1-18), which has complexes that are all of the same shape, size, and direction. It is caused by an ectopic pacemaker site in the ventricle.

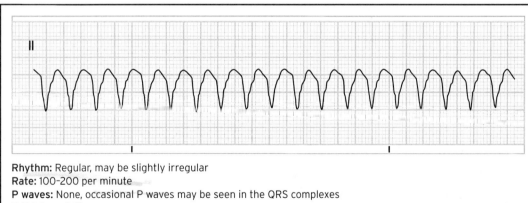

Rhythm: Regular, may be slightly irregular
Rate: 100-200 per minute
P waves: None, occasional P waves may be seen in the QRS complexes
P-R interval: None
QRS complex: Greater than 0.11 seconds, wide and bizarre
P wave to QRS ratio: None

FIGURE 1-18 Monomorphic ventricular tachycardia.

From *Arrhythmia Recognition: The Art of Interpretation*, courtesy of Tomas B. Garcia, MD.

Clinical Significance

Ventricular tachycardia can be the result of many underlying causes, the most common of which are coronary artery disease, Q-T interval prolongation, and electrolyte imbalance, specifically potassium. In ventricular tachycardia, the atria do not contract in their normal synchrony prior to ventricular activation; therefore, the ventricles do not adequately fill with blood before they contract. This can result in a reduction in stroke volume and cardiac output.

In order to initiate ACLS guidelines, the first step is to determine if the ventricular tachycardia is stable or unstable.

Origin: Polymorphic Ventricular Tachycardia

Polymorphic ventricular tachycardia (FIGURE 1-19) has complexes that vary in size, shape, and direction from complex to complex. This dysrhythmia typically occurs when the Q-T interval of the original underlying rhythm becomes prolonged, indicating a severe delay in ventricular repolarization. A variant of polymorphic ventricular tachycardia is torsade de pointes (TdP), which means "twisting of points."

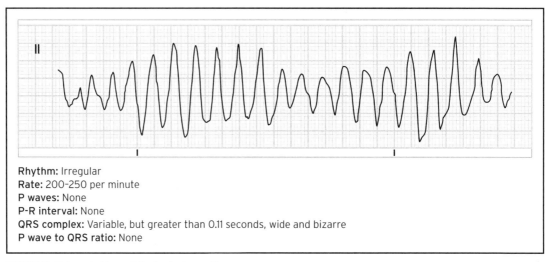

Rhythm: Irregular
Rate: 200-250 per minute
P waves: None
P-R interval: None
QRS complex: Variable, but greater than 0.11 seconds, wide and bizarre
P wave to QRS ratio: None

FIGURE 1-19 Polymorphic ventricular tachycardia.

From *Arrhythmia Recognition: The Art of Interpretation*, courtesy of Tomas B. Garcia, MD.

Clinical Significance

Polymorphic ventricular tachycardia has many of the same causes as its monomorphic counterpart; however, it is particularly prone to occur after the administration of drugs that prolong the Q-T interval. Hypomagnesemia (low blood magnesium level) and hypokalemia (low potassium levels) are commonly associated with polymorphic ventricular tachycardia. Both monomorphic and polymorphic ventricular tachycardias have a high potential for deteriorating to ventricular fibrillation.

Cardiac Arrest Rhythms

Introduction

This section covers the dysrhythmias that do not produce a palpable pulse, leading to cardiac arrest. It is critical to recognize and treat these rhythms as soon as possible to maximize the patient's chance of survival.

Ventricular Fibrillation/Pulseless Ventricular Tachycardia
Origin

Ventricular fibrillation is due to multiple ectopic ventricular pacemakers, which depolarize in a random, chaotic fashion and spread throughout the myocardium. It results in uncontrolled myocardial "quivering" or fibrillating that does not produce cardiac output or a pulse.

Clinical Significance

If untreated, ventricular fibrillation (FIGURE 1-20) is a lethal dysrhythmia. Ventricular fibrillation is the most common initial rhythm in adult sudden cardiac arrest that occurs in a public place. Immediate defibrillation is critical in the management of ventricular fibrillation. Ventricular fibrillation of relatively large amplitude ("coarse") is often initially seen, but becomes less coarse and less responsive to defibrillation as minutes pass. Myocardial ischemia or myocardial infarction is the most common cause of ventricular fibrillation in adults.

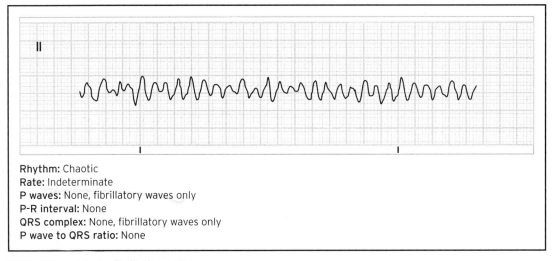

Rhythm: Chaotic
Rate: Indeterminate
P waves: None, fibrillatory waves only
P-R interval: None
QRS complex: None, fibrillatory waves only
P wave to QRS ratio: None

FIGURE 1-20 Ventricular fibrillation (V-fib).

From *Arrhythmia Recognition: The Art of Interpretation*, courtesy of Tomas B. Garcia, MD.

Note

Ventricular tachycardia (V-tach), covered previously in the section on tachycardia, can present with or without a pulse; pulseless V-tach can occur in patients with cardiac arrest. Although not as often as ventricular fibrillation, ventricular tachycardia may be witnessed as the first rhythm in cardiac arrest before it deteriorates to ventricular fibrillation. Pulseless V-tach treatment is the same as ventricular fibrillation: both require immediate defibrillation.

Asystole

Origin

The term asystole (FIGURE 1-21) in cardiac arrest refers to ventricular asystole. Often, if one looks at the monitor closely, there are still P waves and atrial depolarization but no conduction to the ventricles. This results in a total absence of mechanical activity in the myocardium.

Clinical Significance

For obvious reasons, ventricular asystole does not produce a pulse because the ventricles are not beating. It is commonly the result of untreated ventricular fibrillation that eventually "degenerates" to fine V-fib and ventricular standstill/asystole. Other causes of asystole include severe hypoxia, acidosis, or electrolyte abnormalities.

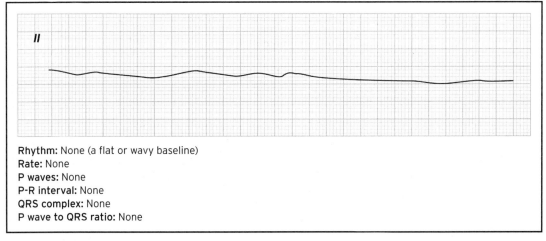

Rhythm: None (a flat or wavy baseline)
Rate: None
P waves: None
P-R interval: None
QRS complex: None
P wave to QRS ratio: None

FIGURE 1-21 Asystole.

From *Arrhythmia Recognition: The Art of Interpretation*, courtesy of Tomas B. Garcia, MD.

Pulseless Electrical Activity (PEA)

PEA is not a particular cardiac rhythm. Rather, it is a condition in which an organized cardiac rhythm is not accompanied by a palpable pulse. PEA can be caused by anything that impedes myocardial mechanical activity or causes profound shock. Treatable causes of PEA include hypoxia, hydrogen ion (acidosis), hypovolemia, hyperkalemia, hypothermia, toxins, tamponade (cardiac), tension pneumothorax, thrombosis (pulmonary), and thrombosis (coronary).

Summary

It is important to evaluate the cardiac rhythm and the patient's signs and symptoms to determine the most appropriate treatment approach.

More than one cardiac rhythm disturbance can be observed in the same patient over a short time period. This requires the clinician to be versatile in changing the course of management very quickly. It is important to analyze and interpret the cardiac rhythm, the full vital signs, and overall patient status. This careful and systematic assessment is also crucial in determining whether the presenting cardiac rhythm is causing hemodynamic compromise.

Pharmacologic and Electrical Therapy

Introduction

This chapter reviews the most common pharmacologic and electrical interventions used in ACLS to treat patients with a variety of cardiovascular emergencies. After a careful and systematic assessment of your patient, you must determine whether pharmacologic or electrical therapy is indicated.

Although many of the medications reviewed in this chapter have standard adult dosages, alterations in those dosages may be required, depending on the patient's hemodynamic status.

Other medications that may not be listed in this text may also be required to treat patients with cardiovascular emergencies.

Acute Coronary Syndrome and Stroke

Introduction

The medications reviewed in this section, which are used to achieve various therapeutic effects, are often indicated in patients who present with signs and symptoms suggestive of an acute coronary syndrome (eg, myocardial infarction, unstable angina) or acute ischemic stroke.

Aspirin (Acetylsalicylic Acid/ASA)

Therapeutic Effects

Aspirin blocks the formation of thromboxane A_2, thus inhibiting platelet aggregation and vasoconstriction. Aspirin reduces overall mortality from acute myocardial infarction and reduces the incidence of reinfarction and nonfatal stroke.

Indications

- Signs and symptoms suggestive of an acute coronary syndrome, such as chest discomfort
- ECG changes that are consistent with acute coronary syndrome, such as ischemic ST-segment depression, T-wave inversion, or ST-elevation consistent with myocardial infarction in a patient with signs and symptoms of acute coronary syndrome.

Contraindications

- Known hypersensitivity to aspirin
- Bleeding disorders (eg, hemophilia)
- Active ulcer disease or recent gastrointestinal bleeding

Adult Dose

- Administer 2 to 4 chewable aspirin (162–324 mg) nonenteric coated as soon as possible after the onset of symptoms. Aspirin suppository (300 mg) is a safe alternative if severe nausea, vomiting, or gastrointestinal disorders are present.
  - To achieve a rapid therapeutic blood level, instruct the patient to chew the aspirin before swallowing.

Fibrinolytic Therapy

Therapeutic Effects

Numerous fibrinolytic agents are on the market, each of which may produce varying mechanisms of action. These drugs produce a therapeutic effect of breaking down the fibrin and fibrinogen matrix of a thrombosis (fibrinolysis), thus fragmenting the clot that is obstructing an artery and reestablishing distal blood flow.

Indications

- Acute myocardial infarction in adults
  - ST-segment elevation in a pattern that is consistent with an MI of greater than or equal to 1 mm in two or more contiguous leads
  - In the context of signs and symptoms of acute myocardial infarction (ie, chest pain) of greater than 15 minutes and less than 12 hours, and PCI is not available within 90 minutes of medical contact
- Acute ischemic stroke (Alteplase is the only fibrinolytic agent approved for use)
  - Sudden onset of focal neurologic deficit (ie, slurred speech, facial droop, hemiparesis or hemiparalysis) or alterations in mental status
  - Absence of intracerebral/subarachnoid hemorrhage (ruled out with head computed tomography [CT])
  - Signs and symptoms not rapidly improving (ie, transient ischemic attack)
  - Signs and symptoms of 3-hour duration and of no greater than 4.5-hour duration in carefully selected patients

Exclusion Criteria for Fibrinolytic Therapy

- Systolic BP >180 to 200 mm Hg diastolic or >100 to 110 mm Hg on presentation
- Right versus left arm systolic BP difference >15 mm Hg
- History of structural central nervous system disease
- Significant closed head or facial trauma within the previous 3 months
- Ischemic stroke >3 hours or <3 months EXCEPT for acute ischemic stroke being considered for fibrinolytic therapy
- Recent (within 2 to 4 weeks) major trauma or surgery (including laser eye surgery)
- Gastrointestinal/genitourinary bleeding
- Prior intracranial hemorrhage
- Bleeding disorder or internal bleeding (including <2 to 4 weeks)
- Active bleeding (including menses)
- Current anticoagulant use (ie, warfarin [Coumadin])
- Pregnancy
- Serious systemic disease (ie, advanced cancer, severe liver or kidney disease)

Adult Dose

- Variable, depending on the fibrinolytic agent used

Morphine Sulfate (MSO$_4$)

Therapeutic Effects

Morphine is a narcotic analgesic that promotes, through its vasodilatory effects, systemic venous pooling of blood, which reduces venous return to the heart (preload) as well as systemic vascular resistance (afterload). By this mechanism, morphine is effective in reducing myocardial oxygen demand and consumption. Additionally, its narcotic analgesic effect reduces chest discomfort and anxiety. Administration of morphine should be reserved for treatment of ischemic chest pain refractory to nitrate therapy.

Not responding to GTN

Indications

- Chest discomfort in acute coronary syndrome that is not completely relieved by nitroglycerin
- Cardiogenic pulmonary edema (with a systolic blood pressure greater than 90 mm Hg)

Contraindications

For patients with unstable angina (UA/NSTEMI), caution is advised due to large registry findings of potentially adverse effects of morphine and an association with increased mortality.

- Hypersensitivity to morphine or other opiate drugs
- Signs of central nervous system depression (eg, respiratory depression, bradycardia, hypotension)

Adult Dose

- 2- to 4-mg increments via slow IV push given over 1–5 minutes. The dose may be repeated every 5–30 minutes as needed to achieve the desired effect.
  - Should signs of central nervous system (CNS) depression occur, naloxone (Narcan) may need to be given in a dose of 0.4 to 2 mg via IV to reverse this effect.

Nitroglycerin (NTG)

Therapeutic Effects

Nitroglycerin, which is a nitrate, is a smooth muscle relaxant that produces systemic venous pooling of blood through its vasodilatory effects. This effect decreases venous return to the heart (preload) as well as systemic vascular resistance (afterload), which may result in decreased myocardial oxygen consumption.

Indications

- Chest discomfort suspected to be of cardiac origin
- Cardiogenic pulmonary edema secondary to left-sided heart failure

Contraindications

Extreme caution is advised in administering nitrates to a patient with acute STEMI of inferior wall. Right-sided ECG must be checked for right ventricular infarction (RVI).

- Systolic blood pressure of less than 90 mm Hg or greater than 30 mm Hg below baseline
- Severe bradycardia (<50 beats/min) or tachycardia (>100 beats/min) in the absence of heart failure
- Use of sildenafil (Viagra), avanafil (Stendra), or vardenafil (Levitra, Staxyn) within the past 24 hours
- Use of tadalafil (Cialis, Adcirca) within the past 48 hours

Adult Dose

- Sublingual tablets: 0.4 mg (1 tablet) repeated in 5-minute intervals to a maximum of three tablets
- Sublingual spray: 1 spray (0.4 mg metered dose) repeated in 5-minute intervals to a maximum of three sprays
- IV infusion: 10–20 mcg/min titrated to desired effect
  - Frequently monitor the blood pressure (BP).

Oxygen (O₂)

Therapeutic Effects

Oxygen increases hemoglobin saturation and enhances tissue oxygenation, provided that adequate ventilation and circulation are maintained.

Indications

- Oxygen saturation level less than or equal to 94%
- Confirmed or suspected hypoxemia
- Ischemic chest pain
- Respiratory insufficiency
- Prophylactically during air transport

- Confirmed or suspected carbon monoxide poisoning
- All other causes of decreased tissue oxygenation
- Decreased level of consciousness

Contraindications
- None, when given in emergency situations

Dose and Method of Administration (Regardless of Age)
- Titrate to maintain an SpO_2 level of greater than 94%.
- When a bag-mask device is in use, administer at 15 L/min.

Antiarrhythmics

Introduction
Antiarrhythmic medications are used to treat a variety of cardiac arrhythmias, both supraventricular (narrow complex) and ventricular (wide complex) in origin. The medications reviewed in this section are addressed in eACLS.

Adenosine (Adenocard)
Therapeutic Effects
Cardioversion with adenosine is very quick and effective with minimal and transient side effects. Adenosine is a naturally occurring (endogenous) nucleoside that is rapidly metabolized. Adenosine slows the discharge rate of the SA node and slows conduction through the AV node. It is often given to try to restore a normal sinus rhythm in patients with PSVT by terminating reentry through the AV node, or to transiently slow AV conduction so the type of tachycardia can be determined more easily.

Indications
Adenosine may be useful in differentiating SVT from V-tach and in converting wide complex tachycardia of supraventricular origin. Adenosine should be considered only if the rhythm is regular and the QRS is monomorphic.
- Narrow QRS complex supraventricular tachycardias (ie, supraventricular tachycardia [SVT]) to slow the ventricular rate and determine the underlying rhythm
- In PSVT to attempt termination

Contraindications
- Toxin-induced tachycardias
- Second- or third-degree atrioventricular (AV) block
- Obvious atrial fibrillation/flutter
- Ventricular tachycardia

Do not use adenosine in patients with known Wolff-Parkinson-White syndrome and irregular polymorphic wide complex tachycardia.

Adult Dose
- Initial dose
  - 6-mg rapid (over 1–3 seconds) IV/IO push administered through the access site that is closest to the heart with the extremity elevated, followed immediately by a 20-mL saline flush
- Repeat dose
  - 12 mg via rapid IV push 1–2 minutes after initial dose, immediately followed by a 20-mL saline flush, if needed

Dose Variations
- Larger doses may be needed in the setting or high blood level or theophylline, caffeine, or theobromine.
- Lower initial dose of 3 mg may be used in patients taking dipyridamole or carbamazepine, those with transplanted hearts, or if given by central venous access.
- Caution: Side effects with adenosine are common but transient. Flushing, dyspnea, and chest discomfort are observed most frequently.

Amiodarone (Cordarone)
Therapeutic Effects
Amiodarone is an antiarrhythmic drug with diverse electrophysiologic effects. It is a multichannel blocker (ie, sodium, potassium, calcium channel, and alpha and beta blocker) that prolongs AV conduction, AV refractory period and QRS and Q-T intervals, thereby slowing the heart rate. Amiodarone is the first-line antiarrhythmic agent for cardiac arrest because it has been clinically shown to improve the rate of ROSC and hospital admission in adults with refractory V-fib/pulseless V-tach. Amiodarone may be considered when V-fib/V-tach is unresponsive to CPR, defibrillation, and vasopressor therapy. Amiodarone is particularly useful for slowing conduction in the His-Purkinje system and in accessory pathways of patients with Wolff-Parkinson-White (WPW) syndrome.

Indications
- Stable irregular narrow complex tachycardia (atrial fibrillation)
- Stable regular narrow complex tachycardia
- To control rapid ventricular rate due to accessory pathway conduction in pre-excited atrial arrhythmias
- Hemodynamically stable monomorphic V-tach
- Polymorphic V-tach with normal Q-T interval
- V-fib and pulseless V-tach that is refractory to defibrillation or reoccurs
- Wide complex tachycardia of uncertain origin
- Stable V-tach when cardioversion is successful
- Adjunct to synchronized cardioversion in supraventricular tachycardias (eg, atrial tachycardia)
- Termination of ectopic atrial tachycardia
- Rate control in atrial fibrillation and atrial flutter when other therapies prove ineffective

Contraindications
Use caution when administering with other drugs that prolong Q-T (ie, procainamide)
- Known sensitivity to amiodarone
- Cardiogenic shock
- Sinus bradycardia
- Sinus node disease with resultant significant bradycardia
- Second- and third-degree AV block

WARNING: Amiodarone infusion rate should be decreased if there is a significant drop in blood pressure (due to its vasodilatory effects), prolongation of the Q-T interval, or heart block. Stop the infusion if the QRS widens to >50% of baseline or hypotension develops. Other potential complications of amiodarone include bradycardia and torsade de pointes. Amiodarone should not be administered together with another conduction blocking agent.

Adult Dose
- V-fib and pulseless V-tach
  - 300 mg diluted in 20–30 mL of D₅W via rapid IV push
  - Repeat dose of 150 mg diluted in 20–30 mL of D₅W via rapid IV push 3–5 minutes after the initial dose
- Stable V-tach, SVT, and atrial flutter/fibrillation
  - 150 mg (3 mL of amiodarone added to 100 mL of D₅W) infused over 10 minutes
    - You may repeat this dose every 10 minutes as needed.
- 24-hour maintenance infusion
  - 1 mg/min infusion for 6 hours (360 mg)
  - Then 540 mg via IV infusion over the remaining 18 hours (0.5 mg/min)
  - Maximum dose: 2.2 grams in 24 hours

Lidocaine (Xylocaine)

Therapeutic Effects

Lidocaine blocks the influx of sodium through the fast channels of the myocardium, which suppresses ventricular arrhythmias, but not as effectively.

Indications

- Cardiac arrest V-fib, and pulseless V-tach that is refractory to defibrillation
  - Used as an alternative to amiodarone if not available
- Stable wide complex tachycardias (eg, V-tach, wide complex tachycardias of uncertain origin)
- Hemodynamically stable monomorphic V-tach

Contraindications

- Known hypersensitivity to lidocaine or "caine" type medications (eg, Novocain)
- Sinus bradycardia
- Atrioventricular blocks

Adult Dose

- V-fib and pulseless V-tach
  - 1–1.5 mg/kg via rapid IV/IO push
    - A single dose of 1.5 mg/kg is acceptable in cardiac arrest.
    - Repeat doses can be given at 1–1.5 mg/kg via rapid IV push every 8–10 minutes to maximum cumulative dose of 3 mg/kg.
- Stable V-tach and wide complex tachycardia of uncertain origin
  - 1–1.5 mg/kg via rapid IV/IO push
  - Repeat 0.5–0.75 mg/kg every 5–10 minutes to a maximum total dose of 3 mg/kg.
- Maintenance infusion
  - 1–4 mg/min titrated to desired effect

Magnesium Sulfate (MgSO$_4$)

Therapeutic Effects

Officially classified as an electrolyte, magnesium possesses antiarrhythmic-like properties. Magnesium slows the impulse rate of the SA node and suppresses automaticity in partially depolarized cells. Magnesium produces vasodilation and may cause hypotension if administered rapidly.

Indications

- Polymorphic V-tach (eg, torsade de pointes [TdP]) with a pulse
- Cardiac arrest only if hypomagnesemia is present and polymorphic V-tach is displaying on the cardiac monitor
- Severe refractory V-fib, after other antiarrhythmics have proven unsuccessful
- Ventricular arrhythmias due to digitalis toxicity

Contraindications

- CNS depression
- Hypermagnesemia
- Hypocalcemia

Adult Dose

- Polymorphic V-tach (torsade de pointes) with a pulse
  - Loading dose of 1–2 g mixed in 10 mL of D$_5$W, given via IV over 5–60 minutes
  - Follow with 0.5–1 g/hour IV for up to 24 hours, titrated to control torsade de pointes.
  - Cardiac arrest from hypomagnesemia or torsade de pointes
    - 1–2 g (2–4 mL of a 50% solution) diluted in 10 mL of D$_5$W, given via IV over 5–20 minutes

Caution: Side effects include hypotension, CNS depression, and respiratory depression, particularly in those with renal impairment

Procainamide (Pronestyl)

Therapeutic Effects

Procainamide slows conduction in the atria, ventricles, and His-Purkinje system by prolonging the P-R and Q-T intervals and the refractory period of the AV node. Procainamide slows the refractory period within the atria and ventricles, and slows the conduction velocity.

Indications

- Stable SVT that is refractory to vagal maneuvers or treatment with adenosine
- Stable wide complex tachycardias of uncertain origin
- Atrial fibrillation with a rapid ventricular rate in patients with WPW   *Wolf Parkinson White*
- V-fib and pulseless V-tach that is refractory to defibrillation and other antiarrhythmics

Contraindications

- Avoid in patients with Q-T prolongation and CHF.
- Known sensitivity to procainamide or similar medications
- Third-degree AV block
- Digitalis toxicity (may exacerbate AV conduction depression)
- Preexisting prolongation of the QRS complex and Q-T intervals

Adult Dose

- Recurrent V-fib and pulseless V-tach
  - 20 mg/min via IV infusion
    - 100 mg via rapid IV push every 5 min is acceptable in cardiac arrest.
  - In urgent situations, up to 50 mg/min may be administered.
    - The use of procainamide in cardiac arrest is limited by the need for slow infusion and uncertain efficacy.
  - Total maximum dose: 17 mg/kg
- SVT, atrial fibrillation, and wide complex tachycardia of uncertain origin
  - 20 mg/min via IV infusion
- Maintenance infusion
  - 1–4 mg/min titrated to desired effect
- Stop procainamide infusion when at least one of the following occurs:
  - Arrhythmia suppression
  - Hypotension develops
  - QRS complex widens by greater than 50% of its pretreatment width
  - Maximum dose of 17 mg/kg has been given

Calcium Channel Blockers

Introduction

Calcium channel blockers are used in the treatment of stable narrow complex tachycardias as well as for rate control in atrial fibrillation and atrial flutter.

Diltiazem (Cardizem)   *use if β Blockers CI or ise Rective BNF*
Therapeutic Effects

Prophylaxis
of Rx for Angina
↓ Hypertension

Diltiazem blocks the movement of calcium ions across the cell membranes of the myocardium and smooth muscles of the vasculature. This effect results in decreased myocardial contractility (negative inotropy), slowing of conduction through the AV node (negative dromotropy), and dilation of the coronary arteries and peripheral vasculature, which decreases myocardial oxygen demand and may result in lower blood pressure.

Indications

- Control of the ventricular rate in atrial fibrillation, atrial flutter, and reentry supraventricular tachycardias
- Adjunct to adenosine to treat stable narrow complex tachycardias

Contraindications

- Hypotension
- Cardiogenic shock
- Wide complex tachycardias of uncertain origin
- Poison- or drug-induced tachycardias
- Rapid atrial fibrillation, and atrial flutter in patients with WPW
- AV heart block (without an artificial pacemaker)
- Concurrent administration of beta-blocking drugs (eg, Atenolol®, Inderal®) particularly if given via IV
  - May precipitate significant hypotension

Adult Dose

- IV bolus
  - 15–20 mg (0.25 mg/kg) IV over 2 minutes
    - You may repeat 15 minutes later at 20–25 mg (0.35 mg/kg) over 2 minutes.
  - Maintenance infusion
    - 5–15 mg/hour, based on the initial dose needed to control the rate

Electrical Therapy

Introduction

Electrical therapy is used frequently in emergency treatment for patients who have serious signs and symptoms as a result of their cardiac rhythm. Serious signs and symptoms include acutely altered mental status, ischemic chest discomfort, acute heart failure, hypotension, or other signs of shock. Patients whose heart rates are too slow, too fast, or chaotic and without a pulse need electrical therapy to stabilize their condition.

Defibrillation

Therapeutic Effects

Defibrillation is the unsynchronized delivery of energy into the myocardium. The therapeutic effect of defibrillation is to depolarize all the cardiac cells at once, so an organized cardiac pacemaker (eg, SA or AV node) can restore a perfusing rhythm.

Indications

- V-fib or pulseless V-tach, unstable polymorphic V-tach
- Early defibrillation is the single most important therapy for V-fib and pulseless ventricular tachycardia (V-tach), and should be initiated without delay.

Contraindications

- Asystole
  - Routine defibrillation of asystole is not recommended, as it may result in failure to identify and treat the underlying cause of asystole.
- Regular cardiac rhythms with a pulse
- Other health care providers are in contact with the patient.
  - You must ensure that nobody is in contact with the patient prior to performing defibrillation.

Adult Energy Settings[1]

- V-fib and pulseless V-tach
  - 120–200 J biphasic or 360 J monophasic
  - Follow each shock immediately with CPR, starting with chest compressions.
  - If the first defibrillation fails to convert V-fib or pulseless V-tach, defibrillate one time, as needed, after every 2 minutes of CPR.
- Unstable polymorphic V-tach
  - 120–200 J biphasic or 360 J monophasic
  - Be prepared to perform CPR if the patient becomes pulseless.

---

[1] Manufacturer recommendation (120–200 J); if unknown, use the maximum available. Second and subsequent doses should be equivalent, and higher doses may be considered.

Synchronized Cardioversion

Therapeutic Effects

Synchronized cardioversion is the timed delivery of energy into the myocardium to correct rapid, regular cardiac rhythms in patients who are hemodynamically unstable as a result of the cardiac rhythm. The device synchronizes the shock delivery when it senses an R wave. This avoids delivering the shock during the relative refractory period (down slope of the T wave), which may increase the likelihood of precipitating V-tach or V-fib.

Indications

- Perfusing narrow and wide QRS complex tachycardias (rate >150 per minute) with serious signs and symptoms linked to the tachycardia (ie, monomorphic V-tach, SVT, atrial fibrillation, atrial flutter)

Contraindications

- V-fib, pulseless V-tach, or polymorphic V-tach (requires defibrillation)
- Certain poison- or drug-induced tachycardias
  - Treat the underlying problem with an antidote, if available.
- Other health care providers are in contact with the patient.

Adult Energy Settings[2]

- Narrow QRS and regular: 50–100 J
- Narrow QRS and irregular: 120–200 J biphasic or 200 J monophasic
- Wide QRS and regular: 100 J
- Wide QRS and irregular: use defibrillation dose 120–200 J biphasic (not synchronized)

Transcutaneous Cardiac Pacing (TCP)

Therapeutic Effects

TCP involves using an artificial electrical impulse to increase the electrical discharge rate of a slow, inherent pacemaker in the heart. TCP is the preferred initial cardiac pacing method in emergency cardiac care because it can be initiated quickly and is relatively safe.

Indications

- Symptomatic bradycardia when the patient's signs and symptoms are linked to the bradycardia and pharmacologic interventions are either unavailable or unsuccessful.
- Examples of cardiac rhythms that may require TCP include:
  - Second-degree type 2 heart block
  - Third-degree heart block

Contraindications

- Severe hypothermia
- Prolonged bradyasystolic cardiac arrest

Adult Energy Settings

- Set the pacing rate at 70 to 80 beats per minute.
  - Symptomatic bradycardia
    - Increase output (mA) from the minimum setting until consistent electrical capture is achieved, as evidenced by a widening of the QRS complex and a broad T wave after each pacer spike.
    - Increase 5 mA further for a safety margin and check pulses for mechanical capture.

Parasympatholytics

Introduction

Also referred to as parasympathetic blockers, vagolytic, and anticholinergic drugs, parasympatholytics block the parasympathetic nervous system via the vagus nerve and are used to treat symptomatic bradycardias (absolute and relative) caused by increased vagal tone. They reverse cholinergic-mediated decreases in heart rate and atrioventricular nodal conduction.

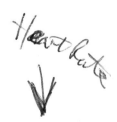

---

[2] Consider administering a short-acting sedative (ie, Midazolam) to the conscious patient before performing cardioversion.

Atropine Sulfate
Therapeutic Effects

By blocking the effects of the acetylcholine on the parasympathetic nervous system, atropine increases the heart rate because it accelerates the discharge rate of the SA node. Atropine also enhances conduction through the atria and the AV node.

Indications

- Hemodynamically unstable bradycardia
- Organophosphate poisoning
- Nerve agent exposure

Contraindications

Use cautiously when bradycardia is due to acute coronary ischemia or MI.

- Tachycardia
- Hypersensitivity
- Unstable cardiovascular status in acute hemorrhage with myocardial ischemia
- Hypothermic bradycardia

Note that atropine may not be effective in treating bradycardia accompanied by second-degree type II and third-degree AV blocks.

Also, in denervated hearts (eg, heart transplant patients), proceed with transcutaneous pacing or catecholamines instead.

Adult Dose

- Symptomatic bradycardia
  - 0.5 mg via rapid IV push
    - Repeat every 3–5 minutes to a maximum dose of 3 mg.
    - Must give rapidly: atropine may cause a paradoxical bradycardia if it is given too slowly.

Sympathomimetics

Introduction

Sympathomimetic drugs mimic the effects of the sympathetic nervous system and are thus used to increase the heart rate and blood pressure. Drugs in this category are usually the synthetically produced equivalent to what is endogenous (naturally occurring) in the human body.

Epinephrine (Adrenalin)
Therapeutic Effects

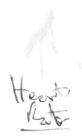

Epinephrine is a naturally occurring catecholamine. It possesses positive alpha and beta adrenergic effects. Its alpha effects result in vasoconstriction, thus increasing the blood pressure. Its selective beta$_1$ effects result in increased heart rate (positive chronotropy) and increased myocardial contractility (positive inotropy). Its selective beta$_2$ effects cause relaxation of bronchial smooth muscle (bronchodilation).

Indications

- Cardiac arrest
  - V-fib/pulseless V-tach, asystole, PEA
- Symptomatic bradycardia
  - If atropine, pacing, and dopamine are ineffective
- Severe hypotension
  - Treat with fluid and boluses first
- Anaphylactic shock
  - Combined with fluid boluses, corticosteroids, and antihistamines

Contraindications

- Tachycardia
- Hypertension
- Hypothermia

- Pulmonary edema
- Myocardial ischemia
- Hypovolemic shock
- Do not mix or infuse simultaneously in the same line with alkaline solutions (eg, sodium bicarbonate), because deactivation of epinephrine, as with all catecholamines, will occur.

Adult Dose

- Cardiac arrest
  - 1 mg (10 mL of 1:10,000 solution) every 3–5 minutes, followed by a 20-mL flush of normal saline IV/IO
  - There is no maximum dose of epinephrine when it is given for persistent cardiac arrest.
- Symptomatic bradycardia or severe hypotension unresponsive to other treatments (ie, fluid boluses, dopamine, etc.)
  - 2–10 mcg/min
    - Add 1 mg of epinephrine (1 mL of 1:1,000 solution) to 250 mL or 500 mL of normal saline.

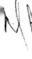

Dopamine (Intropin) 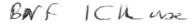 BNF ICU use.

Therapeutic Effects

Dopamine is a naturally occurring catecholamine with alpha and beta adrenergic effects depending on the dose. At low (2 to 5 mcg/kg/min) doses, dopaminergic receptors are stimulated. This causes dilation of the renal and mesenteric arteries. At medium or "cardiac" (5–10 mcg/kg/min) doses, dopamine acts directly on beta$_1$ receptors causing increased myocardial contractility (increased inotropy) and increased heart rate (positive chronotropy). Doses greater than 10 mcg/kg/min (vasopressive dose) stimulate alpha receptors, resulting in an increase in systemic vascular resistance (vasoconstriction). The dosing range of dopamine depends on the patient's clinical condition.

Indications

- Symptomatic bradycardia
  - If atropine, pacing, and epinephrine are ineffective
- Hypotension (systolic BP 70–100 mm Hg) with signs and symptoms of shock
  - Consider fluid boluses first because dopamine should not be given in the setting of intravascular volume depletion.
  - Cardiogenic shock, septic shock, distributive shock

Contraindications

- Known hypersensitivity to dopamine
- Hypovolemia
- Tachydysrhythmias or V-fib
- Pheochromocytoma (an adrenal tumor that produces epinephrine)
- Concurrent use of monoamine oxidase (MAO) inhibitors (ie, Marplan, Parnate, Nardil)
- Do not mix or infuse simultaneously in the same line with alkaline solutions (ie, sodium bicarbonate) because deactivation of dopamine, as with all catecholamines, will occur.

Adult Dose

- As an IV infusion, mix 400–800 mg of dopamine in 250 mL of normal saline, D$_5$W, or lactated Ringer's, and titrate based on the patient's clinical response:
  - Renal protection following resuscitation:
    - 2–5 mcg/kg/min (rarely used in the acute resuscitation phase)
  - Symptomatic bradycardia:
    - 2–10 mcg/kg/min
  - Profound hypotension (non-hypovolemic):
    - 10–20 mcg/kg/min

Vasopressin (Pitressin Synthetic)

Therapeutic Effects

Vasopressin is an antidiuretic hormone (ADH) that is a nonadrenergic vasoconstrictor that causes coronary, renal, and peripheral vasoconstriction.

Indications

- Can be used to replace the first or second dose of epinephrine for patients in cardiac arrest from V-fib/pulseless V-tach, asystole, or PEA

Contraindications

- Known sensitivity to vasopressin
- Acute coronary syndrome
  - Vasopressin may exacerbate hypertension because of its vasoconstrictive effects.

Adult Dose

- 40 units via IV push as a one-time dose

Summary

Selecting the most appropriate emergency intervention for your patient (pharmacologic or electrical) depends on a careful and systematic assessment in order to determine whether the patient is unstable, as evidenced by serious signs and symptoms (eg, chest pain, altered mental state, or shortness of breath). If the patient is unstable, you must determine whether the cardiac rhythm is causing the patient's unstable signs and symptoms or if it is the result of an underlying condition.

When you are preparing to administer a medication, it is important to remember the "six rights" of medication administration, which are:

- **Right** patient
- **Right** drug
- **Right** time
- **Right** dose
- **Right** route
- **Right** documentation

Medication doses and routes may vary, depending on the patient's condition. A particular dose and route for a medication may be therapeutic for one condition but may be detrimental for another.

Digoxin Cardiac Glycoside increases myocardial contraction & reduces conductivity within AV Node. Most useful in controlling Ventricular Response in Atrial flutter & fib.

Hypokalaemia predisposes the Pt to Digitalis toxicity managed by potassium sparing diuretics or suppliments.

Patient Assessment and eACLS Case Review

3

Introduction

The first part of this chapter reviews the general assessment and treatment of patients who are not in cardiac arrest, as well as of patients who are in cardiac arrest. The second part reviews the eight core cases addressed in the eACLS program.

ACLS often provides a general approach to treatment. Additional treatment or variations in treatment may be required, depending on the patient's clinical condition and clinical response to your interventions.

Assessment and Treatment of Non-Cardiac Arrest Patients

Introduction

Successful management of a conscious patient experiencing a cardiovascular or respiratory system emergency requires a careful and systematic assessment of the patient and selection of the appropriate treatment algorithm.

This section reviews the basic assessment and treatment principles specific to patients who are not in cardiac arrest.

Assessing the Patient for Serious Signs and Symptoms

To reduce the likelihood of a cardiac arrest in your patient, you must perform a careful and systematic assessment aimed at identifying serious signs and symptoms linked to their condition or cardiac rhythm (**Table 3-1**). The presence of serious signs and symptoms indicates that your patient is hemodynamically unstable and requires treatment that differs from that of the stable patient.

Table 3-1: Serious Signs and Symptoms

▪ Serious signs
  • Altered mental status
  • Pulmonary edema
  • Jugular venous distention
  • Hypotension
▪ Serious symptoms
  • Chest discomfort or pressure
  • Shortness of breath
  • Dyspnea on exertion

Universal Treatment for the Non-Cardiac Arrest Patient

Certain interventions should be performed on all non–cardiac arrest patients who present with a cardiovascular or respiratory system emergency, regardless of their presenting cardiac rhythm. Table 3-2 reviews those interventions and the reason(s) that they are performed.

Table 3-2: Universal Treatment for the Non-Cardiac Arrest Patient

■ Supplemental oxygen
 • Supplemental oxygen is the first drug administered to spontaneously breathing patients with a cardiovascular or respiratory system emergency if indicated by pulse oximetry.
  – Nasal cannula at 2-6 L/min for patients with mild hypoxia and adequate breathing
  – Nonrebreathing mask at 15 L/min for patients with significant hypoxia
  – Positive-pressure ventilatory support for inadequately breathing patients
■ Pulse oximetry
 • The pulse oximeter indicates gross abnormalities, not subtle changes.
 • Administer oxygen in a concentration that maintains oxygen saturations (SpO_2) of greater than 94%.
■ Cardiac monitoring
 • Cardiac monitoring is an essential assessment tool that is used to identify potentially life-threatening cardiac dysrhythmias.
 • A 12-lead ECG should be obtained to gather additional information regarding your patient's condition.
■ Intravenous therapy
 • An IV line is necessary to administer medications or to give fluid boluses if the patient's blood pressure is low.

Summary

Treating a non–cardiac arrest patient who has a cardiovascular or respiratory system emergency requires a careful and systematic assessment to determine whether the patient is stable or unstable. Your assessment findings will enable you to select the most appropriate treatment for the patient's specific condition.

All patients with a cardiovascular or respiratory system emergency require cardiac monitoring and intravenous therapy. The goal in managing the conscious patient is to prevent cardiac arrest.

Assessment and Treatment of Cardiac Arrest Patients

Introduction

Successful management of a patient in cardiac arrest requires a careful and systematic assessment, immediate identification of the cardiac rhythm, and selection of the appropriate treatment algorithm.

This section reviews the basic assessment and treatment principles specific to patients who are in cardiac arrest.

Assessing the Patient for Underlying Causes of Cardiac Arrest

Patient assessment should include the past medical history and events that preceded the cardiac arrest, to reduce the possibility of missing a potentially reversible underlying cause that is directly linked to the cardiac arrest. Therapies such as defibrillation, epinephrine, and other pharmacologic agents may have minimal or no benefit until the underlying cause can be identified and corrected.

Table 3-3 summarizes the common causes of cardiac arrest, clinical findings suggestive of each cause, and the specific treatment for each cause. The mnemonic "Hs and Ts" will help you

Table 3-3: Underlying Causes of Cardiac Arrest (5 Hs and 5 Ts)

- **Hypovolemia**
  - History of trauma or severe dehydration, flat jugular veins, ECG is rapid with narrow QRS complexes
    - Give a 500-mL bolus of normal saline, and then reassess.
- **Hypoxia**
  - Profound cyanosis, suggestive blood gas readings, airway problems
    - Ensure effective oxygenation and ventilation.
- **Hydrogen ion (acidosis)**
  - History of diabetes (ie, hyperglycemic ketoacidosis), suggestive blood gas readings, bicarbonate-responsive preexisting acidosis, renal failure
    - Ensure effective oxygenation and ventilation first, then consider sodium bicarbonate.
- **Hyperkalemia/hypokalemia**
  - History of renal failure, recent dialysis, diuretic use, and abnormal ECG findings
    - Calcium chloride and sodium bicarbonate for hyperkalemia
    - Cautious infusion of potassium and magnesium for hypokalemia
- **Hypothermia (spontaneous or environmental)**
  - History of recent exposure to cold environment, low core body temperature
    - Remove from the cold environment.
    - Perform active internal rewarming.
    - Limit defibrillations to one attempt and withhold cardiac medications until the core body temperature is raised above 86°F (30°C).
- **Toxins (intentional/accidental overdose [OD])**
  - History of ingestion, empty bottles at the scene, abnormal neurologic exam, bradycardia, tachycardia, prolonged Q-T interval
    - Intubation, activated charcoal, antidotes specific to ingestion (naloxone for narcotics and sodium bicarbonate for tricyclic antidepressants), and hemodialysis for certain agents
- **Tamponade (cardiac)**
  - History of thoracic trauma or invasive cancer, pulses not palpable during CPR, jugular venous distention
    - Pericardiocentesis
- **Tension pneumothorax**
  - History of thoracic trauma, pulses not palpable during CPR, jugular venous distention, absent breath sounds on the affected side, decreased compliance when ventilating, and contralateral tracheal shift (late)
    - Needle decompression (thoracentesis)
- **Thrombosis (coronary, ACS)**
  - History suggestive of acute myocardial infarction (AMI), ST-segment and T-wave changes
    - PCI or fibrinolytics
- **Thrombosis (pulmonary)**
  - Sudden onset of dyspnea, pleuritic chest discomfort, cyanosis before arrest, pulses not palpable during CPR, jugular venous distention
  - Anticoagulation fibrinolytics

remember the potentially reversible underlying causes of cardiac arrest. You should evaluate any patient in cardiac arrest for a potentially reversible cause.

Universal Treatment for the Cardiac Arrest Patient

There are certain interventions that must be carried out in all cases of cardiac arrest, *regardless* of the presenting cardiac rhythm. **Table 3-4** reviews those interventions and the reason(s) that they are performed.

Post-Cardiac Arrest Resuscitation Management

If return of spontaneous circulation (ROSC) occurs, certain interventions should be performed to reduce the recurrence of cardiac arrest. If the patient rearrests, the chances of a second

Table 3-4: Universal Treatment for the Cardiac Arrest Patient

- **CPR**
  - *High-quality* CPR keeps the heart, brain, and other vital organs perfused until the patient's abnormal cardiac rhythm can be corrected with the appropriate treatment.
    - During CPR: push hard and push fast (at least 2 inches deep), deliver compressions at a rate of at least 100 per minute, allow full recoil of the chest in between compressions, and minimize interruptions in chest compressions (10 seconds or less).
- **Airway management**
  - Manage the airway using basic maneuvers first. If basic maneuvers are ineffective, consider inserting an advanced airway.
    - Placement of an advanced airway is recommended only if it can be accomplished with a minimal (<10 second) interruption in chest compressions, or if you are unable to ventilate by noninvasive means.
    - If an advanced airway is placed, use quantitative waveform capnography. Do NOT hyperventilate the patient.
- **Vascular access**
  - Intravenous (IV) or intraosseous (IO) access needs to be established to administer cardiac drugs and, if needed, fluid boluses (normal saline or lactated Ringer's). The IV and IO routes have shown to be equally effective with regard to the medication's onset of action.
- **Vasopressors**
  - Epinephrine, 1 mg IV or IO, is administered every 3-5 minutes in patients in cardiac arrest and should continue until return of spontaneous circulation (ROSC) occurs.
    - Vasopressin, in a one-time dose of 40 units IV, may be used to replace the first or second dose of epinephrine.
- **Circulation of cardiac drugs**
  - All cardiac drugs must be circulated with effective CPR (push hard and push fast) to deliver the drugs to the central circulation.
- **Identify and correct underlying causes**
  - If a careful assessment of your patient is performed, a potentially reversible cause of the cardiac arrest can be identified and corrected, thus increasing the chances of a successful resuscitation.

successful resuscitation are much lower. Prevention of recurrent cardiac arrest can be maximized by performing the appropriate post-cardiac arrest management (**Table 3-5**).

Summary

When treating a patient in cardiac arrest, you must focus on identifying and correcting the underlying cause of the cardiac arrest. Failure to do so will significantly decrease the likelihood of a successful resuscitation.

Table 3-5: Immediate Post-Cardiac Arrest Management

- Optimize ventilation and oxygenation.
  - Maintain SpO_2 at ≥94%.
  - Manage the airway. If it cannot be managed with basic maneuvers, consider an advanced airway (if not already done).
  - Use quantitative waveform capnography, attempt to maintain $ETCO_2$ at 35-40 mm Hg.
  - Provide 10 to 12 breaths per minute (do NOT hyperventilate).
- Treat hypotension (SBP <90 mm Hg).
  - IV or IO fluid bolus
  - Vasopressor infusion (if refractory to fluid boluses)
    - Epinephrine infusion: 0.1-0.5 mcg/kg/min
    - Dopamine infusion: 5-10 mcg/kg/min
- Consider treatable causes.
- Obtain 12-lead ECG.
- Can the patient follow verbal commands?
  - No: Consider induced hypothermia.
  - Yes: STEMI or high suspicion for AMI?
    - Yes: Coronary reperfusion and advanced critical care
    - No: Advanced critical care

Certain interventions must be performed on all patients in cardiac arrest, regardless of their presenting cardiac rhythm (CPR, airway management, vascular access, vasopressor, circulation of cardiac drugs, and identify and treat the underlying cause). These interventions are aimed at maintaining effective ventilation and circulation until the patient's abnormal cardiac rhythm can be corrected with the appropriate treatment.

The appropriate post-cardiac arrest management prevents the patient from redeveloping cardiac arrest. Patients who redevelop cardiac arrest are more difficult to resuscitate a second time.

eACLS Case Review

Introduction

This section reviews the eight core cases addressed in the eACLS program and is intended to provide you with a review of the assessment and management of patients with cardiovascular emergencies. The following core cases are addressed in the eACLS program:

- Acute coronary syndromes (ACS)
- Asystole
- Bradycardia
- Pulseless electrical activity (PEA)
- Stroke
- Tachycardia: Narrow complex
- Tachycardia: Wide complex
- Ventricular fibrillation

Two additional cases—respiratory arrest and use of the automated external defibrillator (AED)—are also included as enrichment material. However, these are not core cases within the eACLS course.

Remember that a careful and systematic assessment of the patient and selection of the appropriate treatment algorithm are critical aspects of patient care that will maximize the chances of a favorable patient outcome.

eACLS Case 1: Acute Coronary Syndromes (ACS)

Introduction

eACLS Case 1 focuses on the assessment and management of the patient who presents with an acute coronary syndrome (ACS), which is a term used to describe either unstable angina or acute myocardial infarction (AMI). The classic symptom of ACS is chest discomfort; however, some patients may have other symptoms more prominent than chest discomfort. It is best to err on the side of treating the patient with chest discomfort as though an acute MI is in progress.

Signs and Symptoms of Acute Coronary Syndrome

A classic symptom of an acute coronary syndrome is chest pain. The patient may describe this pressure as discomfort or heaviness rather than actual pain. This chest pressure or discomfort typically lasts longer than 15 minutes and may or may not be relieved by rest and/or nitroglycerin. Some patients may have more prominent symptoms of nausea; vomiting; epigastric pain; discomfort of the upper body, jaw, and/or neck; dyspnea, sweating, lightheadedness, and dizziness. These atypical symptoms are more common in patients with diabetes, elderly patients, and female patients.

The signs and symptoms of an acute coronary syndrome (Table 3-6) indicate myocardial ischemia. Some patients may present with very few signs and symptoms, whereas others may have many.

Immediate Assessment and Management

Within the first 10 minutes after a patient presents with signs and symptoms of an acute coronary syndrome, an immediate assessment should occur, including ECG and initiation of the appropriate treatment.

> ### Table 3-6: Signs and Symptoms of Acute Coronary Syndrome
>
> - Pressure, squeezing, or discomfort in the center of the chest, generally lasting longer than 15 minutes
>   - May radiate to the shoulders, neck, arms, or jaw, or in the back or between the scapulae
> - Lightheadedness, nausea, or fainting
> - Shortness of breath
>   - May occur without provocation or with exertion
> - Feeling of impending doom

ACS treatment should be initiated at the same time as patient assessment. Treatment is aimed at ensuring adequate oxygenation and ventilation, and relieving pain. The mnemonic "MONA," which stands for **m**orphine, **o**xygen, **n**itroglycerin, and **a**spirin, lists the immediate interventions for the patient with an ACS. Although MONA does not represent the actual sequence of treatment, it is a useful mnemonic to remember. **Table 3-7** summarizes the sequence of immediate assessment and management for the patient with an ACS. Morphine may not be appropriate for some patients with ACS—the practitioner must assess the risks and benefits before ordering this.

> ### Table 3-7: Immediate Assessment and Management of the Patient with ACS
>
> - Administer supplemental oxygen if indicated per pulse oximetry.
>   - Nasal cannula at 1-4 L/min, or nonrebreathing mask at 15 L/min for more severe cases
>   - Monitor oxygen saturation and maintain above 94%.
> - Administer aspirin, 162-324 mg.
>   - To achieve a rapid therapeutic blood level, instruct the patient to chew the nonenteric coated aspirin before swallowing it.
>   - Aspirin should not be given if the patient has a hypersensitivity to salicylates or a known bleeding disorder (eg, hemophilia).
> - Assess vital signs.
> - Apply the cardiac monitor and obtain 12-lead ECG tracing.
> - Initiate an IV of normal saline.
>   - You should also obtain cardiac serum markers, electrolytes, coagulation studies, complete blood count (CBC), and kidney function panel, if possible.
> - Consider nitroglycerin (NTG) sublingual tablets or spray.
>   - Be aware of the patient's blood pressure and phosphodiesterase type 5 inhibitor drug (eg, Sildenafil) use in the last 24 to 48 hours.
>   - Administer with caution in the presence of inferior wall infarct with right ventricular involvement.
>   - Administer up to three nitroglycerin tablets or spray, 5 minutes apart.
> - Give morphine, 2-4 mg via slow IV push.
>   - If three NTG treatments fail to completely relieve the patient's chest discomfort, administer morphine, provided that there are no contraindications and the benefits outweigh the risks.

Targeted History for Fibrinolytic Therapy

Within the first 10 minutes of patient presentation, the patient should undergo ECG, targeted history, and physical exam to assess for eligibility for fibrinolytic therapy. If they are administered within the proper window within the onset of symptoms, fibrinolytic agents, also called "clot busters," can reduce the size of a myocardial infarction, thus preserving cardiac muscle.

Numerous fibrinolytic agents are on the market, and although their individual doses vary, their mechanisms of action are all similar.

The indications, or "inclusion criteria," for fibrinolytic therapy (**Table 3-8**) must be carefully matched to the contraindications, or "exclusion criteria" (**Table 3-9**), because if they are administered to the wrong patient, fibrinolytic agents can be lethal.

Table 3-8: Inclusion Criteria for Fibrinolytic Therapy

- ST-segment elevation consistent with a myocardial infarction (≥1 mm in ≥2 contiguous leads)
  - ST-segment elevation is conclusive only with a 12-lead ECG
- Signs and symptoms of ACS (see **Table 3-6**)
- Onset of symptoms <12 hours ago and PCI is not available within 90 minutes of first medical contact

Table 3-9: Exclusion Criteria for Fibrinolytic Therapy*

- Systolic BP >180 to 200 mm Hg diastolic or >100 to 110 mm Hg on presentation
- Right versus left arm systolic BP difference >15 mm Hg
- History of structural central nervous system disease
- Significant closed head or facial trauma within the previous 3 months
- Ischemic stroke >3 hours or <3 months EXCEPT for acute ischemic stroke being considered for fibrinolytic therapy
- Recent (within 2 to 4 weeks) major trauma or surgery (including laser eye surgery)
- Gastrointestinal/genitourinary bleeding
- Prior intracranial hemorrhage
- Bleeding disorder or internal bleeding (including <2 to 4 weeks)
- Active bleeding (including menses)
- Current anticoagulant use (ie, warfarin [Coumadin])
- Pregnancy
- Serious systemic disease (ie, advanced cancer, severe liver or kidney disease)

*Note: If ANY of the above is present, fibrinolysis MAY be contraindicated.

FIGURE 3-1 represents a 12-lead ECG tracing that indicates an acute anteroseptal wall myocardial infarction (ST-segment elevation in leads $V_1–V_4$) in progress. If the appropriate criteria are met, the patient will benefit from fibrinolytic therapy.

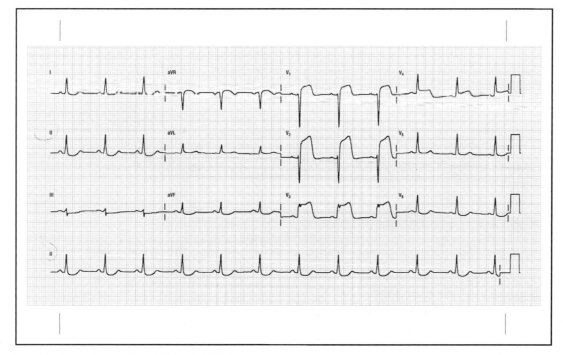

FIGURE 3-1 Acute anteroseptal wall AMI in progress.

From *12-Lead ECG: The Art of Interpretation*, courtesy of Tomas B. Garcia, MD.

Other Reperfusion Strategies

Depending on the patient's presentation and hemodynamic status, other reperfusion strategies may be more appropriate for their condition. Such strategies include percutaneous coronary interventions (PCI), such as a coronary angioplasty with or without stent placement, and coronary artery bypass grafting (CABG).

A careful assessment of the patient's history and hemodynamic status and resources availability determines which reperfusion intervention is most appropriate.

Summary

The patient with signs and symptoms of an acute coronary syndrome requires immediate care. Parameters such as 12-lead electrocardiography, cardiac serum marker analysis, and a brief targeted history with emphasis on potential fibrinolytic candidacy are essential.

Immediate management is aimed at ensuring adequate oxygenation and ventilation and administering pharmacologic interventions to reduce pain and anxiety.

Based on 12-lead ECG findings and a careful assessment of the patient, the most appropriate reperfusion strategy can be selected. The adage "time is muscle" definitely applies and should be remembered when treating the patient with an acute coronary syndrome. If the patient is not assessed and managed within a short period of time, areas of myocardial ischemia or injury could enlarge. This could lead to cardiogenic shock (pump failure), which has a high mortality rate.

eACLS Case 2: Asystole

Introduction

eACLS Case 2 focuses on the assessment and management of the patient in asystole. Asystole represents a total absence of both cardiovascular electrical and mechanical activity on the cardiac monitor, thus producing a "flat line" (FIGURE 3-2). Unfortunately, asystole is rarely associated with a positive outcome.

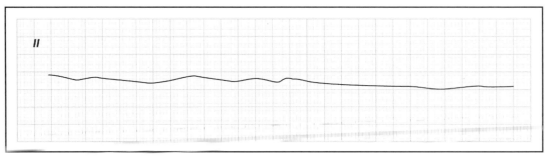

FIGURE 3-2 Asystole.

From *Arrhythmia Recognition: The Art of Interpretation,* courtesy of Tomas B. Garcia, MD.

Treatment for Asystole

After verification of cardiac arrest and confirmation of asystole, you should consider assessing another lead, because asystole in one lead may actually be fine V-fib in another. Treatment of the patient (**Table 3-10**) in asystole requires CPR, airway management, the appropriate medications, and a careful assessment to determine why the patient developed cardiac arrest.

Summary

There are, however, potentially reversible causes of asystole; therefore, a careful and systematic assessment, in addition to treating the cardiac arrest with the appropriate interventions, will maximize the chances of a successful resuscitation.

Table 3-10: Treatment for Asystole

- Confirm cardiac arrest.
  - Begin CPR and apply the ECG monitor/defibrillator as soon as possible.
- Evaluate the cardiac rhythm.
  - Confirm asystole.
    - Check another lead.
- Continue CPR with minimal interruptions.
- Manage the airway using basic maneuvers first. If basic maneuvers are ineffective, consider inserting an advanced airway.
  - Placement of an advanced airway is recommended only if it can be accomplished with a minimal (<10 second) interruption in chest compressions, or if you are unable to ventilate by noninvasive means.
- Establish vascular access (IV or IO).
- Administer epinephrine, 1 mg (10 mL) of a 1:10,000 solution via rapid IV/IO push every 3-5 minutes.
  - Vasopressin, in a one-time dose of 40 units, can be used to replace the first or second dose of epinephrine.
- Evaluate for and treat the underlying cause of asystole.
  - 5 Hs and 5 Ts
- Consider termination of resuscitative efforts.
  - The determination to cease resuscitative efforts should be based on the following:
    - Was acceptable basic life support (BLS) continued throughout the arrest?
    - If indicated, was an advanced airway device placed and successfully maintained?
    - If present, was V-fib defibrillated?
    - Was vascular access (eg, IV or IO) established?
    - Were all rhythm-appropriate drugs administered?
    - Were potentially reversible causes ruled out or corrected?
    - Has the patient's family been updated on the situation and apprised of the probable negative outcome of continued resuscitation?

---

eACLS Case 3: Bradycardia

Introduction

eACLS Case 3 focuses on the assessment and management of the patient who presents with unstable bradycardia. A careful and systematic assessment must be performed to determine whether serious signs and symptoms linked to the bradycardia are present.

Bradycardia can take on many forms, including sinus bradycardia (FIGURE 3-3) and varying degrees of AV heart block, such as complete (third-degree) heart block (FIGURE 3-4). However, the important concept to remember is that regardless of the rhythm, if the rate is too slow, and the patient is symptomatic as a result of the slow rate, then the bradycardia should be treated.

Bradycardia

Absolute bradycardia exists when the ventricular rate is less than 60 beats per minute. Relative bradycardia exists when the patient's heart rate is slower than one would expect for his or her condition, yet the patient is unstable. For example, a patient with a heart rate of 65 beats per minute and a blood pressure of 80/50 mm Hg may be experiencing a "relative" bradycardia because the pulse rate relative to the blood pressure is too slow.

Treatment for Bradycardia

Treatment for a bradycardic rhythm depends on the presence or absence of serious signs and symptoms. The asymptomatic patient may require little more than close monitoring; however, the unstable patient requires interventions aimed at increasing the heart rate and improving perfusion (Table 3-11).

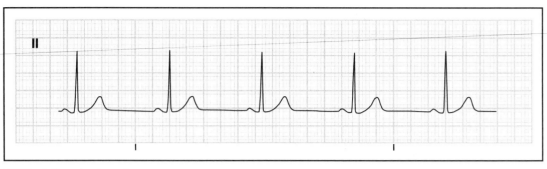

FIGURE 3-3 Sinus bradycardia.

From *Arrhythmia Recognition: The Art of Interpretation*, courtesy of Tomas B. Garcia, MD.

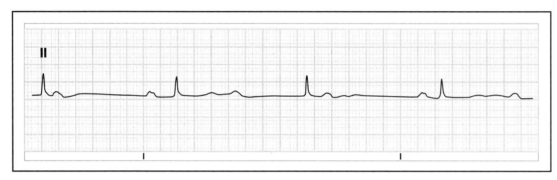

FIGURE 3-4 Third-degree AV block.

From *Arrhythmia Recognition: The Art of Interpretation*, courtesy of Tomas B. Garcia, MD.

Table 3-11: Treatment for Unstable Bradycardia

- Initiate an IV line of normal saline.
- 12-lead ECG
  - A 12-lead ECG may provide more information regarding the patient's condition.
- Interventions aimed at increasing the heart rate may include:
  - Atropine, 0.5 mg via rapid IV push
    - Patients with denervated hearts, such as those who have undergone a heart transplant, are not likely to respond to atropine and require immediate transcutaneous pacing (TCP).
  - TCP
    - Immediate TCP should be initiated for patients with second-degree type II and third-degree.
  - Epinephrine infusion at 2-10 mcg/min
  - Dopamine infusion at 5-10 mcg/kg/min
    - Consider a normal saline bolus before giving dopamine.

Summary

The patient with bradycardia who is asymptomatic generally requires little more than monitoring. However, for the patient presenting with serious signs and symptoms linked to the bradycardia, immediate interventions aimed at increasing the heart rate are indicated.

The patient may require treatment of "relative bradycardia" if the heart rate is over 60 beats per minute but the heart rate is inappropriately low for the patient's condition (ie, low blood pressure or decreased level of consciousness). This requires the same interventions as the patient with absolute bradycardia.

eACLS Case 4: Pulseless Electrical Activity (PEA)

Introduction

eACLS Case 4 focuses on the assessment and management of a patient who presents with pulseless electrical activity (PEA), which is characterized by a rhythm on the cardiac monitor when the patient does not have a detectable pulse. Virtually any cardiac rhythm can be seen in conjunction with PEA. The only exception to this is V-fib and pulseless V-tach, both of which are treated with immediate defibrillation and are not managed as PEA.

Treatment for PEA

In addition to managing the cardiac arrest itself (**Table 3-12**), a critical aspect in managing the patient with PEA is to focus on identifying and treating the underlying cause of the cardiac arrest. Refer to **Table 3-3** for the common causes of cardiac arrest, their clinical signs, and their respective treatments. As a general rule, rhythms that are slow indicate hypoxia, and rhythms that are fast indicate hypovolemia.

Table 3-12: Treatment for PEA

- Confirm cardiac arrest.
  - Begin CPR and apply the ECG monitor/defibrillator as soon as possible.
- Evaluate the cardiac rhythm.
- Continue CPR.
- Manage the airway. Consider inserting an advanced airway if basic maneuvers are not effective.
- Establish vascular access (IV or IO).
  - Consider giving a 500-mL normal saline bolus, even without specific evidence of hypovolemia.
    - Hypovolemia is a common and potentially reversible cause of PEA.
- Administer epinephrine, 1 mg via rapid IV/IO push every 3-5 minutes.
  - Vasopressin, in a one-time dose of 40 units, may be used to replace the first or second dose of epinephrine.
- Evaluate for and treat the underlying cause of PEA.
  - Hs and Ts
- Consider sodium bicarbonate, in special resuscitation scenarios only (ie, hyperkalemic arrest, tricyclic antidepressant overdose), not for routine use in cardiac arrest.
  - The initial treatment of acidosis—regardless of the underlying cause—is to ensure adequate oxygenation and ventilation.

Summary

Any rhythm can deteriorate into PEA. Close attention must be given to the patient's pulse, blood pressure, and underlying condition.

Treatment for PEA involves treating the cardiac arrest with CPR, airway management, IV therapy, and medications. The ultimate goal is to identify and treat the underlying cause of the cardiac arrest rapidly.

eACLS Case 5: Stroke

Introduction

eACLS Case 5 focuses on the assessment and management of the patient with an acute ischemic stroke. An ischemic stroke is the result of a blocked cerebral artery. Common causes include the formation of a local thrombus (**FIGURE 3-5**) or a thrombus that breaks free (embolus) and travels to the brain from another part of the body (**FIGURE 3-6**). Less common causes of acute stroke include cerebral hemorrhage, arterial vasospasm, or generalized hypoperfusion (shock).

All areas distal to the blocked artery are deprived of oxygen, resulting in varying degrees of neurologic impairment ranging from limited mobility to total debilitation.

Stroke Survival and Recovery

When caring for a stroke patient, the goal is to be able to begin therapy no more than 60 minutes from arrival at the hospital door and within 3 hours, and within 4.5 hours for carefully selected patients. This requires that both prehospital and hospital providers avoid any delays.

The 7 Ds of stroke survival and recovery (**Table 3-13**) represent pivotal points during the assessment and care for the stroke patient in which the highest potential for delay exists.

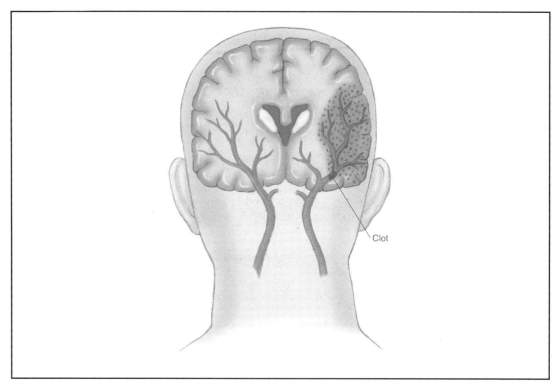

FIGURE 3-5 Thrombotic stroke.
© Jones & Bartlett Learning

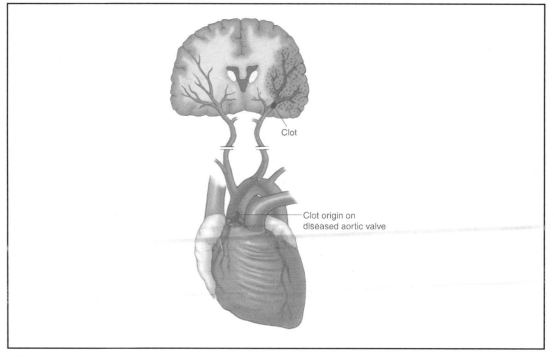

FIGURE 3-6 Embolic stroke.
© Jones & Bartlett Learning

Assessment

After assessment and appropriate management of airway, breathing, and circulation, a rapid assessment of the patient and a brief, targeted history help you identify the patient's potential for having a stroke, enabling prompt treatment. The warning signs of an acute ischemic stroke include:

- Confusion
- Slurred speech (dysarthria)

Table 3-13: The 7 Ds of Stroke Survival and Recovery

- **D**etection of stroke symptoms
- **D**ispatch of EMS in a prompt manner
- **D**elivery of prehospital care and transport by paramedics
- **D**oor-to-treatment time no longer than 60 minutes
- **D**ata collected by the physician after examining the patient
- **D**ecision to begin specific stroke treatment (ie, fibrinolytics, intra-arterial strategies)
- **D**rug administration (or intra-arterial strategy) as soon as the decision has been made

---

- Unilateral facial droop
- Unilateral weakness or paralysis

It is particularly important to determine when the symptoms began. If the patient meets the inclusion criteria, fibrinolytic therapy can be initiated; however, this must be accomplished within 3 hours of the onset of symptoms, and within 4.5 hours in carefully selected patients.

Stroke Scales

Two scales used to gauge the severity of a stroke are the National Institutes of Health (NIH) Stroke Scale and the Cincinnati Prehospital Stroke Scale.

The National Institutes of Health Stroke Scale is one of the stroke scales used—mainly by hospital providers. The scale incorporates multiple variables and produces a numerical score that is a marker of a stroke's severity. Important parameters of the NIH stroke scale include a patient's level of consciousness, awareness, and muscle strength.

The Cincinnati Prehospital Stroke Scale is used by hospital and prehospital providers, and is composed of three tests to help assess whether a patient may be having a stroke (**Table 3-14**). An abnormal finding in any one of these three tests indicates a high probability of a stroke.

Treatment

Treatment for the stroke patient is mainly supportive and focuses on protecting the airway and delivering supplemental oxygen, monitoring the ECG, providing IV therapy, and promptly transporting or transferring the patient to a facility that specializes in stroke care, where fibrinolytic therapy can be initiated (**Table 3-15**).

Table 3-14: Cincinnati Prehospital Stroke Scale

- Facial droop
  - Normal: both sides of the face move equally
  - Abnormal: one side of the face does not move
- Arm drift (instruct the patient to close his or her eyes)
  - Normal: both arms move equally
  - Abnormal: one arm drifts compared with the other
- Speech
  - Normal: the patient uses correct words with no slurring
  - Abnormal: the patient slurs words, uses inappropriate words, or is mute

---

Table 3-15: Treatment for the Stroke Patient

- Provide supplemental oxygen.
- Initiate an IV line of normal saline.
- ECG monitoring
  - Certain cardiac dysrhythmias (eg, atrial fibrillation) can cause a stroke.
  - Monitor and treat the patient for cardiac dysrhythmias.
- Transport/transfer the patient for definitive care.
  - A facility that specializes in stroke management can perform a CT scan of the head and initiate fibrinolytic therapy when indicated.

Fibrinolytic Therapy for Acute Ischemic Stroke

If the onset of symptoms of acute ischemic stroke is within 4.5 hours and the patient meets the inclusion criteria (Table 3-16), he or she may be eligible for fibrinolytic therapy. At the present time, alteplase (Activase) is the only fibrinolytic agent approved by the United States Food and Drug Administration (FDA) to treat an acute thrombotic stroke. If this drug is given promptly, neurologic deficit resulting from the stroke can be minimized. Refer to Table 3-9 for fibrinolytic exclusion criteria.

Table 3-16: Fibrinolytic Inclusion Criteria for Acute Thrombotic Stroke

- Sudden onset of the following:
  - Focal neurologic deficits
    - Abnormal stroke scale
  - Alterations in level of consciousness
- Intracranial hemorrhage ruled out with a head CT
- Symptoms not rapidly improving spontaneously

Summary

An acute ischemic stroke can be a catastrophic event that can leave the patient with permanent disabilities, ranging from mild neurologic deficits to complete incapacitation. All patients with a possible acute ischemic stroke require supplemental oxygen, IV therapy, and cardiac monitoring. After a careful and systematic assessment of the patient, the clinician must act quickly, identify the patient as a candidate for fibrinolytic therapy, and transport or transfer the patient for this critical intervention.

When caring for a stroke patient, the goal is to be able to begin therapy no more than 60 minutes from arrival at the hospital door and within 3 hours of the onset of the symptoms, 4.5 hours in carefully selected patients.

eACLS Case 6: Narrow Complex Tachycardia

Introduction

eACLS Case 6 focuses on the assessment and management of the patient who presents with a narrow complex tachycardia. The term narrow complex tachycardia refers to a rhythm in which the QRS complex is less than 0.11 seconds (less than 2.5 small boxes on the ECG graph paper), and a ventricular rate that is >100 beats per minute (FIGURE 3-7).

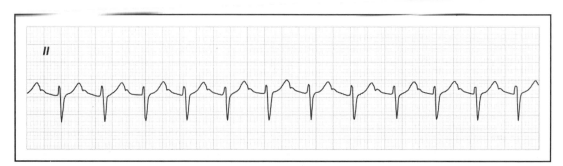

FIGURE 3-7 Narrow complex tachycardia.
From *Arrhythmia Recognition: The Art of Interpretation*, courtesy of Tomas B. Garcia, MD.

Supraventricular tachycardia (SVT) indicates that the origin of the cardiac rhythm is above (supra) the ventricles. SVT can include a variety of different narrow complex tachycardias, such as atrial tachycardia and atrial fibrillation or flutter with a rapid ventricular rate (RVR), among others.

Treatment for Narrow Complex Tachycardia

A careful and systematic assessment must be performed so that the most appropriate treatment can be provided to the patient. If the patient is not experiencing serious signs and symptoms linked to the tachycardia, the initial treatment involves interventions aimed at decreasing the ventricular rate and identifying the underlying cardiac rhythm (Table 3-17).

If serious signs and symptoms are linked to the tachycardia, then synchronized cardioversion (Table 3-18) must be performed without delay. Ventricular rates of less than 150 per minute typically do not require synchronized cardioversion.

Summary

Treatment for the patient with a narrow complex tachycardia requires a careful and systematic assessment in order to identify serious signs and symptoms linked to the tachycardia.

If the patient is stable, initial treatment is aimed at decreasing the heart rate with a combination of vagal maneuvers and pharmacologic interventions, which may enable you to identify the underlying cardiac rhythm and adjust further treatment accordingly.

Unstable patients require immediate synchronized cardioversion, which, in the conscious patient, should be preceded with a sedative agent.

Table 3-17: Treatment for Stable Narrow Complex Tachycardia

- Initiate an IV line of normal saline.
- Obtain a 12-lead tracing.
- Therapeutic interventions aimed at decreasing the heart rate may include:
  - Vagal maneuvers (eg, carotid sinus massage, Valsalva)
  - Adenosine, 6 mg via rapid (over 1-3 seconds) IV push. A second dose of 12 mg adenosine can be given 1-2 minutes later, if needed.
- Pharmacologic interventions
  - Antiarrhythmics
    - Amiodarone, 150 mg IV over 10 minutes (dilute in 100 mL of D_5W), which may be repeated every 10 minutes as needed
  - Calcium channel blockers
    - Diltiazem, 15-20 mg (0.25 mg/kg) IV push over 2 minutes, which may be repeated 15 minutes later at 20-25 mg (0.35 mg/kg) IV push over 2 minutes

---

Table 3-18: Treatment for Unstable Narrow Complex Tachycardia

- Initiate an IV line of normal saline.
- Have suction airway equipment readily available.
- Consider providing short-acting sedation to the conscious patient.
  - Midazolam, 1-2.5 mg via slow IV push
- Ensure that no one is in contact with the patient.
- Push the "sync" button on the defibrillator and verify that the device is syncing.
- Perform synchronized cardioversion.
  - Narrow QRS complex and regular: 50-100 J (If the initial shock fails, increase the dose in a stepwise fashion.)
  - Narrow QRS complex and irregular: 120-200 biphasic J or 200 monophasic J (If the initial shock fails, providers should increase the dose in a stepwise fashion.)

eACLS Case 7: Wide Complex Tachycardia

Introduction

eACLS Case 7 focuses on the assessment and management of the patient with a wide complex tachycardia. A wide complex tachycardia refers to a rhythm in which the QRS complexes are equal to or greater than 0.12 seconds in width and the ventricular rate is greater than 100 beats per minute.

Approximately 90% of wide complex tachycardias are ventricular tachycardia, indicating that the rhythm originated from an ectopic pacemaker in the ventricles. Any wide complex tachycardia should be assumed to be ventricular tachycardia until proven otherwise.

Monomorphic ventricular tachycardia (FIGURE 3-8) has QRS complexes that are all of the same shape and direction. Polymorphic ventricular tachycardia (FIGURE 3-9), a variant of which is torsade de pointes, has QRS complexes that are of varying shapes and direction and resembles a combination of V-tach and V-fib.

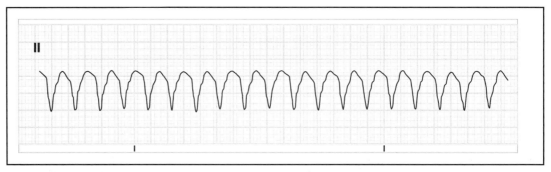

FIGURE 3-8 Monomorphic V-tach.

From *Arrhythmia Recognition: The Art of Interpretation*, courtesy of Tomas B. Garcia, MD.

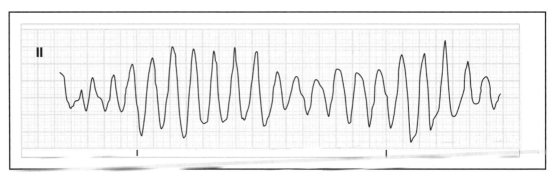

FIGURE 3-9 Polymorphic V-tach.

From *Arrhythmia Recognition: The Art of Interpretation*, courtesy of Tomas B. Garcia, MD.

Treatment for Wide Complex Tachycardias

Wide complex tachycardias (eg, V-tach) have a propensity for deteriorating to ventricular fibrillation and cardiac arrest. It is therefore of great importance that a careful and systematic assessment of the patient is performed to identify serious signs and symptoms linked to the wide complex tachycardia, and the most appropriate treatment algorithm is selected.

If the patient is not experiencing serious signs and symptoms linked to the tachycardia, the initial treatment involves pharmacologic interventions, which are aimed at decreasing ventricular irritability, thus terminating the tachycardia (**Table 3-19**).

If serious signs and symptoms linked to the tachycardia exist, synchronized cardioversion (**Table 3-20**) must be performed without delay. Because of the high risk of deterioration to V-fib, you must be prepared to perform defibrillation if the patient becomes pulseless.

If V-tach is not controlled pharmacologically, proceed with defibrillation.

Table 3-19: Treatment for Stable Wide Complex Tachycardias

- Initiate an IV line of normal saline and obtain a 12-lead ECG.
- Pharmacological interventions may include:
  - Monomorphic V-tach
    - Amiodarone, 150 mg over 10 minutes (diluted in 100 mL of normal saline), which may be repeated every 10 minutes as needed[1]
      - Follow with maintenance infusion of 1 mg/min for the first 6 hours, followed by 0.5 mg/min for the remaining 18 hours; maximum dose of 2.2 g per 24 hours
    - Lidocaine, 1-1.5 mg/kg
      - Repeat 0.5-0.75 mg/kg every 5-10 minutes until the maximum dose of 3 mg/kg has been given.
      - A maintenance infusion of 1-4 mg/min can be considered if the rhythm is terminated.
    - Procainamide, 20 mg/min via IV infusion until any one of the following occurs:
      - Dysrhythmia is suppressed
      - Hypotension develops
      - QRS duration increases by >50% of its pretreatment width
      - Maximum dose of 17 mg/kg has been given
      - A maintenance infusion of 1-4 mg/min can be considered as needed.
  - Polymorphic V-tach (ie, torsade de pointes)
    - Correct electrolyte abnormalities (ie, hypomagnesemia, hyperkalemia)
    - Magnesium sulfate
      - Loading dose of 1-2 g mixed in 10 mL of normal saline or D_5W, over 30-60 seconds
      - Follow with an IV infusion at 0.5-1 g per hour (titrated to control torsade de pointes).
- Electrical interventions as needed (if the patient becomes unstable)

Table 3-20: Treatment for Unstable Wide Complex Tachycardia

- Supplemental oxygen
- Initiate an IV of normal saline.
- Have advanced airway equipment and suction readily available.
- Consider sedation for the conscious patient.
  - Midazolam, 1-2.5 mg via slow IV push
- Push the "sync" button on the monitor/defibrillator.
- Ensure that nobody is touching the patient.
- Perform synchronized cardioversion.
  - 100 monophasic J (or equivalent biphasic); increase the energy setting in a stepwise fashion
    - For unstable polymorphic V-tach with a pulse, defibrillate.[2] Do not attempt cardioversion.
    - Begin CPR if the patient becomes pulseless.

Antiarrhythmic Maintenance Infusions

If a wide complex tachycardia is pharmacologically terminated, begin a maintenance infusion of the antiarrhythmic agent that aided in the conversion (ie, amiodarone, procainamide).

If synchronized cardioversion was used to terminate the wide complex tachycardia and an antiarrhythmic agent was not administered, give a bolus of an antiarrhythmic and begin a maintenance infusion.

It is important to maintain a therapeutic blood level of the appropriate antiarrhythmic agent because this may prevent the recurrence of the wide complex tachycardia. Refer to the chapter on pharmacologic and electrical therapy for the appropriate antiarrhythmic maintenance infusion doses.

Summary

When a patient presents with a wide complex tachycardia, you should assume that it is V-tach until proven otherwise. Continuous hemodynamic monitoring of the patient is essential because wide complex tachycardias can deteriorate to V-fib.

---

[1] Consider adenosine only if regular and monomorphic.

[2] If the patient becomes pulseless or develops V-fib, turn off the synchronizer and defibrillate immediately.

All patients with wide complex tachycardias require IV therapy and cardiac monitoring. A 12-lead ECG may provide additional information regarding the wide complex tachycardia. Treatment is based on whether the patient is stable or unstable; therefore, the clinician must perform a careful and systematic assessment to identify serious signs and symptoms linked to the wide complex tachycardia. Stable wide complex tachycardias are treated with medication; unstable rhythms are treated with electricity (cardioversion or defibrillation depending on the rhythm).

eACLS Case 8: Ventricular Fibrillation

Introduction

eACLS Case 8 focuses on the assessment and advanced management (electrical and pharmacologic) of the patient with V-fib or pulseless V-tach. Basic management of these dysrhythmias is reviewed in eACLS Case 9: Automated External Defibrillation.

It is important to reiterate that for every minute V-fib or pulseless V-tach persists, the patient's chance of survival is reduced by 7% to 10%. The single most important treatment for V-fib (FIGURE 3-10) or pulseless V-tach (FIGURE 3-11) is rapid defibrillation (monophasic or biphasic equivalent).

Treatment for V-Fib and Pulseless V-Tach

The treatment algorithm for V-fib and pulseless V-tach (Table 3-21) assumes that the patient's condition remains unchanged. The clinician must be prepared to quickly change to the appropriate treatment algorithm on the basis of the patient's clinical response to therapy.

Summary

V-fib and pulseless V-tach are lethal dysrhythmias that do not produce a pulse. V-fib is the most common initial dysrhythmia in cardiac arrest, and if it is not treated promptly, it will deteriorate to asystole.

Successful management requires a rapid assessment to confirm cardiac arrest. Begin CPR and apply the cardiac monitor/defibrillator as soon as possible. If V-fib or pulseless V-tach is present, ensure that nobody is touching the patient, deliver one shock, and immediately resume CPR (starting with chest compressions).

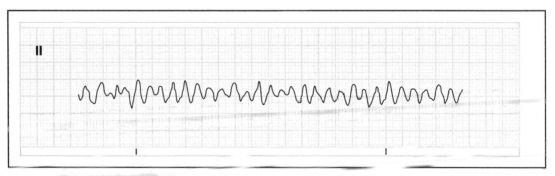

FIGURE 3-10 Ventricular fibrillation.
From *Arrhythmia Recognition: The Art of Interpretation*, courtesy of Tomas B. Garcia, MD.

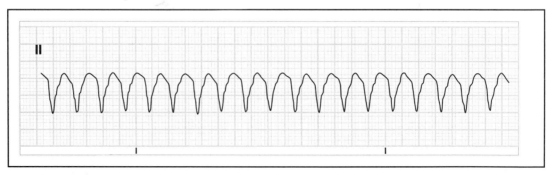

FIGURE 3-11 Ventricular tachycardia.
From *Arrhythmia Recognition: The Art of Interpretation*, courtesy of Tomas B. Garcia, MD.

Table 3-21: Treatment for V-Fib and Pulseless V-Tach

- Confirm pulselessness and apnea.
- Start CPR, give oxygen, and apply the monitor/defibrillator as soon as possible.
- Evaluate the cardiac rhythm.
  - Ensure that nobody is touching the patient.
  - Deliver one shock.
  - *Immediately* resume CPR, starting with chest compressions.
- Perform CPR for 2 minutes (30:2 compression-to-ventilation ratio).
- Establish IV or IO access.
  - Administer epinephrine, 1 mg every 3-5 minutes, via rapid IV/IO push.
    - Vasopressin, in a one-time dose of 40 units, may be used to replace the first or second dose of epinephrine.[3]
- Reassess the rhythm after 2 minutes of CPR.
  - Deliver one shock, if indicated, and immediately resume CPR starting with chest compressions.
- Manage the airway. Consider inserting an advanced airway device if basic maneuvers are ineffective.
  - Use waveform capnography.
  - Perform CPR; deliver at least 100 compressions/min; give one breath every 6-8 seconds (8-10 breaths/min); minimize interruptions in CPR.
- Reassess the rhythm after 2 minutes of CPR.
  - Deliver one shock, if indicated, and *immediately* resume CPR starting with chest compressions.
- Administer amiodarone, 300 mg via rapid IV/IO push.
  - You may repeat one time in 5 minutes at 150 mg.[4]

Further management includes establishing IV or IO access and administering the appropriate pharmacologic agents. Manage the airway with basic maneuvers. If these are ineffective, consider inserting an advanced airway device. Use quantitative waveform capnography to confirm and monitor correct advanced airway placement.

Perform CPR for 2 minutes and then reassess the patient's cardiac rhythm and, if necessary, his or her pulse. Defibrillate again, if needed, and immediately resume CPR (starting with chest compressions). Deliver at least 100 compressions per minute and avoid unnecessary interruptions in CPR.

eACLS Case 9: Automated External Defibrillation (AED)

Introduction

eACLS Case 9 focuses on the management of cardiac arrest with the automated external defibrillator (AED). Most adult cardiac arrest patients present with ventricular fibrillation (V-fib) as the initial cardiac dysrhythmia. V-fib does not produce a pulse; therefore, blood is not circulated throughout the body. Pulseless ventricular tachycardia, although less common, is just as lethal as V-fib.

The single most important treatment for these lethal ventricular dysrhythmias is early defibrillation. When effective, defibrillation "stuns" the heart, causing momentary asystole, thus allowing a dominant cardiac pacemaker to restore organized electrical activity and a perfusing rhythm.

V-fib is a transient rhythm and eventually deteriorates to asystole without prompt defibrillation. The AED can provide rapid defibrillation and does not require an ALS provider to operate.

The simplistic functionality of the AED requires little on the part of the rescuer other than turning on the machine and following the directions of the AED's voice prompt.

After a brief period of analysis, the AED determines whether the patient is in a "shockable" rhythm (eg, V-fib or pulseless V-tach) and informs the rescuer that a shock is advised.

---

[3] Circulate all drugs with high quality CPR for 2 minutes, followed by defibrillation as needed. Following defibrillation, immediately resume CPR (starting with chest compressions) and reassess in 2 minutes.

[4] Lidocaine, 1–1.5 mg/kg (max. dose of 3 mg/kg) may be given as an alternative to amiodarone.

Assessment and Initial Management

A quick assessment of the patient (SKILL 3-1) is required to recognize cardiac arrest. Establish unresponsiveness. Check for breathing by briefly scanning the chest for movement. If breathing is adequate, place the patient in the recovery position and monitor. If the patient is

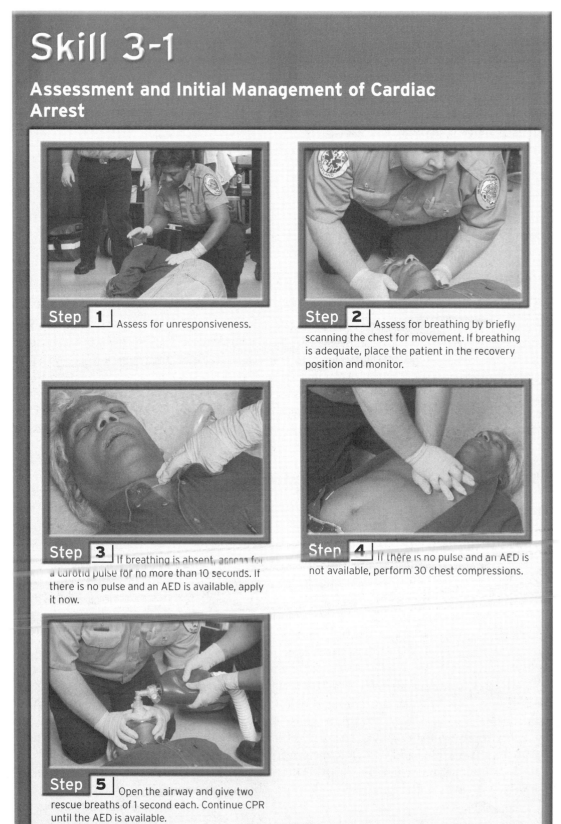

Skill 3-1

Assessment and Initial Management of Cardiac Arrest

Step **1** Assess for unresponsiveness.

Step **2** Assess for breathing by briefly scanning the chest for movement. If breathing is adequate, place the patient in the recovery position and monitor.

Step **3** If breathing is absent, assess for a carotid pulse for no more than 10 seconds. If there is no pulse and an AED is available, apply it now.

Step **4** If there is no pulse and an AED is not available, perform 30 chest compressions.

Step **5** Open the airway and give two rescue breaths of 1 second each. Continue CPR until the AED is available.

unresponsive and is not breathing (or has agonal gasps), assess for a carotid pulse for no more than 10 seconds. If a pulse is present, but the patient is not breathing, open the airway and perform rescue breathing. If there is no pulse and an AED is available, apply it now. If there is no pulse and an AED is not available, begin CPR and apply the AED as soon as it is available.

Cardiac Rhythm Analysis and Defibrillation

As soon as the AED is available, it should be attached to the patient without delay (SKILL 3-2). According to the American Heart Association, for each minute that V-fib or pulseless V-tach persists, the patient's chance of survival is reduced by approximately 7% to 10%.

If the AED detects a shockable rhythm during its analysis, it will indicate that a shock is advised and will prompt the rescuer to deliver a shock. After shock delivery, immediately perform CPR. After two minutes of CPR, the AED will advise to reanalyze the cardiac rhythm. If another shock is advised, deliver the shock and immediately resume CPR (starting with chest compressions). If no shock is advised, resume CPR (starting with chest compressions).

Summary

A rapid patient assessment is required in order to confirm the presence of cardiac arrest and begin the appropriate treatment as soon as possible.

After confirming that a patient is in cardiac arrest, begin CPR and apply the AED as soon as it is available. For one- and two-rescuer adult CPR, use a compression to ventilation ratio

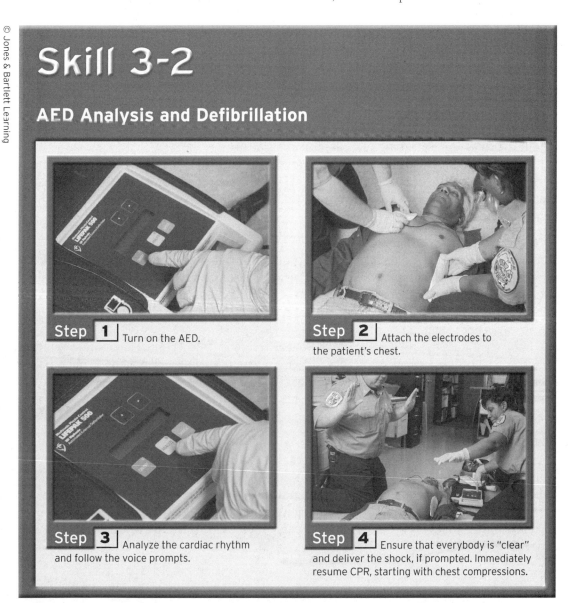

Skill 3-2

AED Analysis and Defibrillation

Step 1 Turn on the AED.

Step 2 Attach the electrodes to the patient's chest.

Step 3 Analyze the cardiac rhythm and follow the voice prompts.

Step 4 Ensure that everybody is "clear" and deliver the shock, if prompted. Immediately resume CPR, starting with chest compressions.

of 30:2. Deliver compressions at a rate of at least 100 per minute and allow the chest to fully recoil in between each compression. Minimize interruptions in CPR and switch compressor roles every 2 minutes.

Failure to recognize and immediately treat V-fib or pulseless V-tach usually results in rapid deterioration to asystole, in which the chance of successful resuscitation is minimal.

eACLS Case 10: Respiratory Arrest

Introduction

eACLS Case 10 focuses on the assessment and management of the patient with respiratory arrest, including respiratory arrest caused by a foreign body airway obstruction (FBAO). You must perform a rapid assessment of the patient to identify the presence of respiratory arrest. Immediate positive-pressure ventilations must then be provided, while maintaining airway patency. Failure to recognize and treat the apneic patient immediately can lead to cardiopulmonary arrest and death of the patient.

Assessment

If a patient is not breathing (as evidenced by a lack of chest movement), but has a pulse, you should open the airway and ensure that it is clear of secretions or obstructions. In the noninjured patient, this is accomplished by performing the head tilt-chin lift maneuver, or the jaw-thrust maneuver in the patient with a suspected spinal injury. It should be noted, however, that if the jaw-thrust maneuver does not open the patient's airway effectively, the head tilt-chin lift maneuver should be performed. It is critical to maintain a patent airway at all times; if vomitus or other secretions are in the airway, they must be removed with suction immediately.

Management

Initial management for the patient in respiratory arrest involves maintaining a patent airway with a combination of manual positioning of the head, and the insertion of a basic airway adjunct, such as an oropharyngeal or nasopharyngeal airway.

Positive-pressure ventilations are then provided with a bag-valve mask or a pocket mask device at a rate of 10–12 breaths per minute (1 breath every 5–6 seconds). You must ensure that supplemental oxygen is attached to the ventilatory device you are using to deliver high concentrations of oxygen.

Foreign Body Airway Obstruction (FBAO)

A foreign body, such as a piece of food, can obstruct the airway and prevent the patient from moving air. FBAO is suspected when there is airway resistance and/or a lack of chest rise when the airway is open and attempts are made to ventilate. Clearly, this is a dire emergency that must be corrected immediately. Further management of the patient would clearly be futile if the airway is not patent.

If the chest does not rise visibly and/or there is resistance during initial attempts to ventilate the patient, reposition the patient's head, and then reattempt to ventilate. If breaths do not produce visible chest rise, perform 30 chest compressions to attempt to dislodge the obstruction (SKILL 3-3).

If chest compressions fail to dislodge the airway obstruction, visualize the vocal cords with a laryngoscope (direct laryngoscopy), and remove the obstruction with Magill forceps (SKILL 3-4).

Advanced Airway Management

While there are many advanced airway devices that you can utilize to secure a patient's airway, endotracheal intubation (SKILL 3-5) provides the best protection against aspiration if the patient regurgitates. Patients in both respiratory and cardiac arrest usually require prolonged ventilatory support and are at an increased risk for regurgitation and aspiration of stomach contents; therefore, you should secure their airway with an endotracheal tube or another advanced airway device.

Preoxygenation of the patient using a bag mask or a pocket mask device for 2 to 3 minutes is a crucial step before intubation is performed. Preoxygenation provides the patient with pulmonary oxygen reserve because ventilations are interrupted during the intubation procedure.

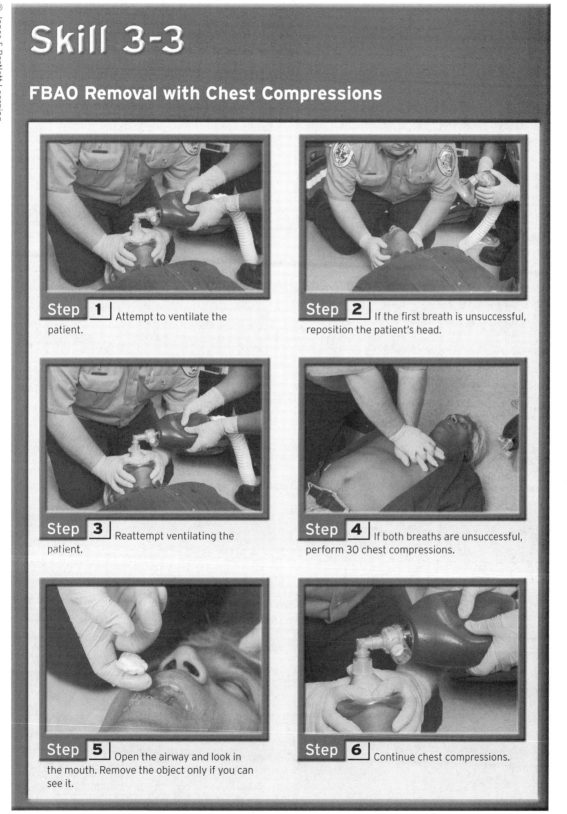

Skill 3-3

FBAO Removal with Chest Compressions

Step 1 Attempt to ventilate the patient.

Step 2 If the first breath is unsuccessful, reposition the patient's head.

Step 3 Reattempt ventilating the patient.

Step 4 If both breaths are unsuccessful, perform 30 chest compressions.

Step 5 Open the airway and look in the mouth. Remove the object only if you can see it.

Step 6 Continue chest compressions.

Skill 3-4

FBAO Removal with Magill Forceps

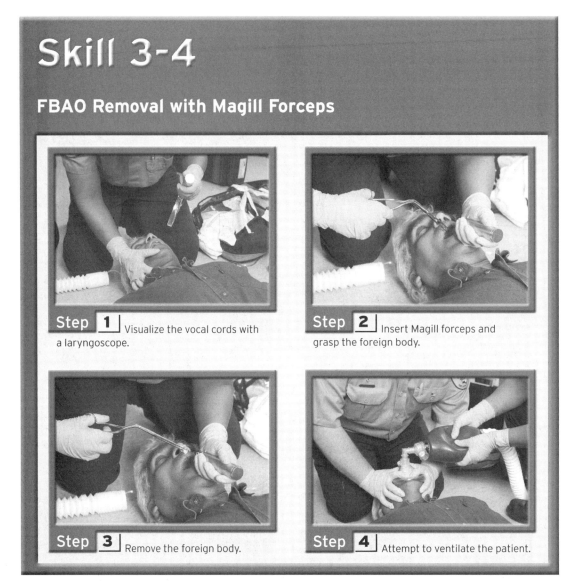

Step 1 Visualize the vocal cords with a laryngoscope.

Step 2 Insert Magill forceps and grasp the foreign body.

Step 3 Remove the foreign body.

Step 4 Attempt to ventilate the patient.

Skill 3-5

Performing Endotracheal Intubation

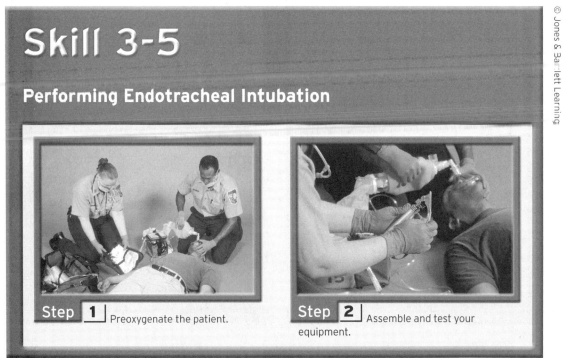

Step 1 Preoxygenate the patient.

Step 2 Assemble and test your equipment.

Continues

Skill 3-5

Performing Endotracheal Intubation, continued

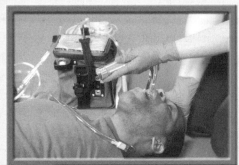

Step 3 Insert the laryngoscope and visualize the vocal cords.

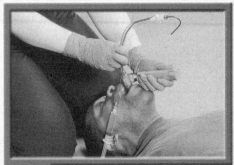

Step 4 Advance the tube to the proper depth in between the vocal cords.

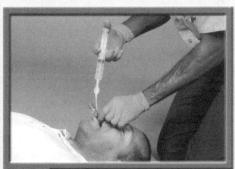

Step 5 Inflate the distal cuff with 5–10 mL of air and disconnect the syringe.

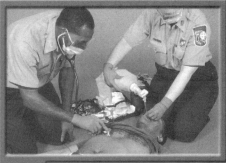

Step 6 Ventilate the patient, confirm correct tube placement by auscultating over both lungs and the epigastrium, and attach an end-tidal CO_2 detector. Waveform capnography should be used to confirm initial tube placement and to monitor ongoing tube position.

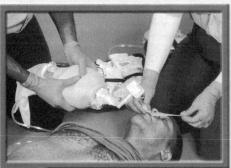

Step 7 Properly secure the tube and continue to ventilate.

Alternative Airway Devices

If endotracheal intubation is unsuccessful, and basic airway management techniques do not provide adequate ventilation, alternative airway devices may be available that enable you to secure a patent airway.

The laryngeal mask airway (LMA) is inserted blindly into the airway while it is guided in place with the middle finger (FIGURE 3-12). The mask, when properly seated, covers the esophagus and facilitates air flow into the lungs.

Dual-lumen airway devices, such as the esophageal Combitube (FIGURE 3-13), are also acceptable alternatives to intubation. Dual-lumen devices are advanced blindly into the airway and come to rest in the esophagus in most cases. Verification of placement is accomplished by ventilating into the tube that produces clear and equal breath sounds and no epigastric sounds and confirmed with waveform capnography.

Other alternative advanced airway devices, such as the King LT, and supraglottic airway devices (ie, CobraPLA), can also be used as alternatives to endotracheal intubation.

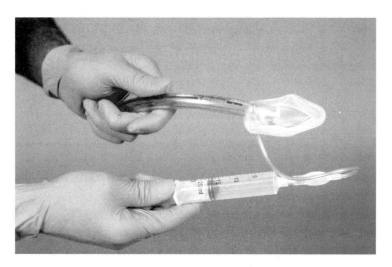

FIGURE 3-12 The laryngeal mask airway.
© Jones & Bartlett Learning

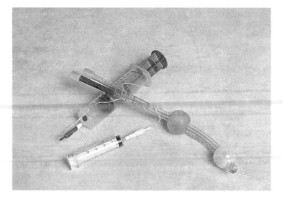

FIGURE 3-13 Esophageal Combitube.
© Jones & Bartlett Learning

Summary

Before assessing the patient's breathing, you must first ensure that the airway is open and clear of obstructions. After confirming the absence of breathing, provide two ventilations with a bag-mask or a pocket mask device.

If initial ventilations are unsuccessful, a foreign body airway obstruction is likely, and corrective action should be taken to relieve the obstruction. This involves chest compressions initially, and removal of a foreign body, if necessary, with Magill forceps under direct laryngoscopy.

Once the airway is patent, continue positive-pressure ventilations. Consider inserting an advanced airway device for patients who require prolonged ventilatory support.

4

eACLS Practice Cases

Introduction

This chapter of the eACLS course manual presents 10 practice cases that are designed to prepare you for the interactive case simulations in the eACLS program. The practice cases are arranged randomly, thus requiring you to identify the patient's cardiac rhythm, to determine whether the patient is stable or unstable, and to administer the appropriate treatment.

For each practice case, pertinent patient assessment information, including chief complaint, ECG rhythms, vital signs, and physical exam findings, is provided. This assessment information will enable you to answer the treatment-related questions that are asked throughout the case.

Questions with a higher degree of difficulty will be labeled "**Beyond eACLS Basics**" and are intended to assess a more in-depth knowledge of the patient's condition. A summary, which contains the answers and rationales to the case questions, follows each respective practice case.

eACLS Practice Case 1

A conscious and alert 50-year-old man complains of a sudden onset of palpitations and lightheadedness, which began approximately 30 minutes previously. Currently, the patient denies chest discomfort or shortness of breath. The pulse oximeter reads 92% on room air.

Question 1: What initial treatment is indicated for this patient?

The initial treatment for this patient is complete. As your assistant prepares to initiate an IV line of normal saline, you attach the ECG leads to the patient's chest and assess his cardiac rhythm (FIGURE 4-1).

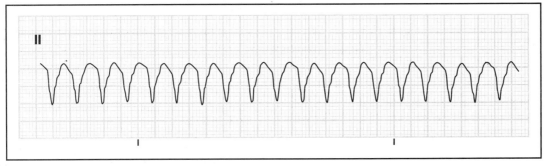

FIGURE 4-1 Your patient's cardiac rhythm.

From *Arrhythmia Recognition: The Art of Interpretation*, courtesy of Tomas B. Garcia, MD.

Question 2: What is your interpretation of this cardiac rhythm?

The patient's blood pressure is 138/78 mm Hg. The pulse is 182 BPM and is strong, and respirations are 20 breaths per minute and unlabored. Further assessment reveals that the patient's breath sounds are clear and equal bilaterally, and his jugular veins are normal. Your assistant reports that the IV line is patent and running at a keep-vein-open (KVO) rate.

Question 3: What treatment is indicated for this patient's condition?

You have just performed the appropriate intervention for the patient's condition when you note a marked decrease in his level of consciousness. You immediately reassess his blood pressure, which is 80/50 mm Hg. His skin is diaphoretic, and his breathing is labored. He is placed on a nonrebreathing mask at 15 L/min.

Question 4: How will you treat this patient now?

The patient's condition remains unchanged after your next intervention; however, you repeat the intervention and note a change in his cardiac rhythm (FIGURE 4-2).

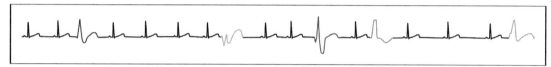

FIGURE 4-2 Your patient's cardiac rhythm has changed.

From *Arrhythmia Recognition: The Art of Interpretation*, courtesy of Tomas B. Garcia, MD.

An immediate reassessment of the patient reveals that his mental status has improved. His blood pressure is 130/70 mm Hg, and his respirations are 18 breaths per minute and unlabored. You prepare to initiate a treatment that is aimed at preventing a recurrence of his dysrhythmia.

Question 5: What will prevent a recurrence of his dysrhythmia?

The patient remains conscious and alert, and his vital signs are stable. His cardiac rhythm now reveals a normal sinus rhythm. With continuous monitoring, you transfer the patient for continued care.

Beyond eACLS Basics

What specific treatment would be required if this patient's potassium level were severely low (less than 2 mEq/L)?

eACLS Practice Case 1 Summary

Question 1: What initial treatment is indicated for this patient?

The patient's oxygen saturation is 92% on room air; therefore, supplemental oxygen via a nasal cannula at 2 to 4 L/min would be appropriate.

Oxygen is indicated if the patient's oxygen saturation is below 94% or if other signs of hypoxemia are present, such as cyanosis or altered mental status. Give a concentration of oxygen that is sufficient to maintain an oxygen saturation of greater than 94%.

Question 2: What is your interpretation of this cardiac rhythm?

The cardiac rhythm depicted is monomorphic V-tach (FIGURE 4-3). The rhythm is regular with a rate of approximately 180 beats per minute. The QRS complexes are wide and bizarre, and there are no discernible P waves. The term "monomorphic" means that all of the QRS complexes are the same size, shape, and direction.

V-tach indicates the presence of an irritable ectopic focus in the ventricles that has become the dominant cardiac pacemaker. If not treated promptly, V-tach could deteriorate to V-fib and cardiac arrest.

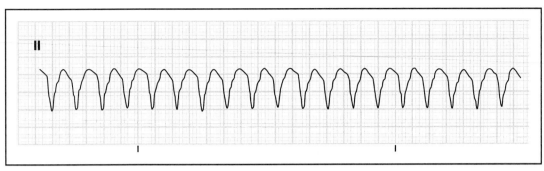

FIGURE 4-3 Your patient's cardiac rhythm.

From *Arrhythmia Recognition: The Art of Interpretation*, courtesy of Tomas B. Garcia, MD.

Question 3: What treatment is indicated for this patient's condition?

This patient is not exhibiting serious signs and symptoms that are linked to his V-tach; therefore, he is considered stable. Treatment with an antiarrhythmic agent is appropriate at this point. Any one of the following medications can be administered:

- Amiodarone: 150 mg over 10 minutes (diluted in 100 mL of normal saline), which may be repeated every 10 minutes as needed
- Lidocaine: 1–1.5 mg/kg
  - Repeat 0.5–0.75 mg/kg every 5–10 minutes until the maximum dose of 3 mg/kg has been given.
- Procainamide: 20 mg/min, via IV infusion
  - The chapter on pharmacologic and electrical therapy discusses further dosing information.

Question 4: How will you treat this patient now?

This patient's condition has clearly taken a turn for the worse. His altered mental status, hypotension, and labored respirations are serious signs and symptoms that indicate hemodynamic instability. After sedating the patient with 2.5 mg of midazolam, you must perform immediate synchronized cardioversion starting with 100 joules. If needed, repeat cardioversion at 200, 300, and 360 joules (70, 120, 150, 200 J on some devices).

Question 5: What treatment will prevent recurrence of his dysrhythmia?

This patient is now in a sinus rhythm with multifocal premature ventricular complexes (PVCs), which indicates continued ventricular irritability and the risk of recurrent V-tach (FIGURE 4-4). An antiarrhythmic maintenance infusion will help to prevent recurrent V-tach. A bolus dose (see previously mentioned doses) must be given before beginning a maintenance infusion. Any one of the following can be used:

- Amiodarone: 360 mg for the first 6 hours (1 mg/min), followed by 540 mg for the remaining 18 hours (0.5 mg/min); the maximum cumulative dose is 2.2 g in 24 hours
- Lidocaine: 1–4 mg/min titrated to the desired effect
- Procainamide: 1–4 mg/min titrated to the desired effect

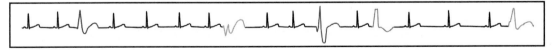

FIGURE 4-4 Your patient's cardiac rhythm has changed.

From *Arrhythmia Recognition: The Art of Interpretation*, courtesy of Tomas B. Garcia, MD.

Beyond eACLS Basics: What specific treatment would be required if this patient's potassium level were severely low (less than 2 mEq/L)?

Normal serum potassium levels range from 2.5 to 5 mEq/L. Potassium levels that are less than 2 mEq/L are often associated with QRS widening, ventricular dysrhythmias, PEA, and asystole.

Specific treatment for hypokalemia-induced V-tach includes the administration of potassium chloride (KCl). Begin the initial infusion at 2 mEq/min over 10 minutes (20 mEq total), followed by 1 mEq/min over the next 10 minutes (10 mEq total). The infusion should be reduced carefully when the patient's condition improves.

eACLS Practice Case 2

A 45-year-old female presents with shortness of breath and nausea that began 45 minutes earlier. She is conscious but confused. You palpate her radial pulse and find that it is slow and weak. After placing her on supplemental oxygen, you assess her cardiac rhythm (FIGURE 4-5).

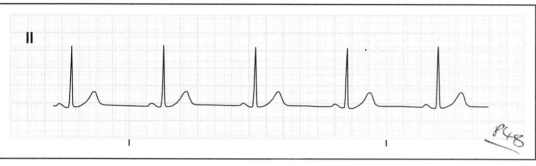

FIGURE 4-5 Your patient's cardiac rhythm.
From *Arrhythmia Recognition: The Art of Interpretation*, courtesy of Tomas B. Garcia, MD.

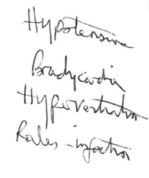

Your patient has a blood pressure of 78/56 mm Hg, a pulse rate of 48 beats per minute weak and regular, and respirations of 24 breaths per minute and labored. Her breath sounds reveal scattered rales bilaterally. An IV line of normal saline is initiated and set at a KVO rate.

Question 1: What pharmacologic agent is indicated for this patient?
The patient's condition remains unchanged, despite receiving the maximum dose of the indicated pharmacologic agent. Your assistant urgently turns your attention to the patient's cardiac rhythm, which has changed (FIGURE 4-6).

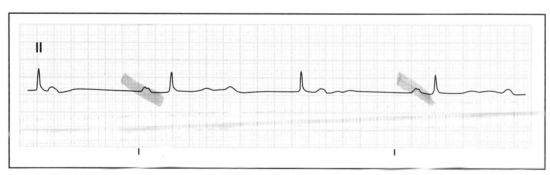

FIGURE 4-6 Your patient's current cardiac rhythm.
From *Arrhythmia Recognition: The Art of Interpretation*, courtesy of Tomas B. Garcia, MD.

Question 2: What intervention is indicated for your patient at this point?
Your next intervention has improved the patient's cardiac rhythm (FIGURE 4-7). Her pulse rate corresponds with the heart rate of her cardiac rhythm.

Although her cardiac rhythm has been corrected, the patient remains hypotensive. After a 500-mL bolus of normal saline fails to increase her blood pressure, you consider the next treatment option.

Question 3: What medication is indicated first for nonhypovolemic hypotension?
The patient's blood pressure is now 108/68 mm Hg, and her pulse rate is 84 beats per minute and strong. She is conscious and alert, and the pulse oximeter reads 98% on the supplemental oxygen.

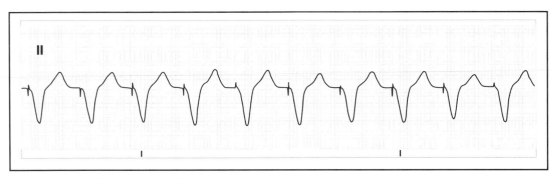

FIGURE 4-7 Your patient's cardiac rhythm has improved.

From *Arrhythmia Recognition: The Art of Interpretation*, courtesy of Tomas B. Garcia, MD.

Question 4: What other medication could have been used to treat this patient's hypotension?

The patient's condition continues to improve. You transfer her for more definitive care while carefully monitoring her cardiac rhythm and vital signs.

Beyond eACLS Basics

How would your treatment have differed had this been a heart transplant patient?

eACLS Practice Case 2 Summary

Question 1: What pharmacologic agent is indicated for this patient?

The patient is displaying sinus bradycardia with a rate of approximately 50 beats per minute. The rhythm is accompanied by serious signs and symptoms such as shortness of breath, hypotension, and an altered mental status, all of which her slow heart rate is causing. The first pharmacologic agent indicated for her condition is atropine sulfate 0.5 mg via a rapid IV push, which may be repeated every 3 to 5 minutes to a maximum vagolytic dose of 3 mg.

Question 2: What intervention is indicated for your patient at this point?

Your patient is now in a third-degree AV block, which represents total AV dissociation (**FIGURE 4-8**). The treatment of choice for this cardiac rhythm is TCP, which serves as a bridge device until a transvenous pacemaker can be inserted or a permanent pacemaker can be implanted. Note that atropine may not be effective in treating bradycardia accompanied by second-degree type II or third-degree AV block; TCP is a more appropriate initial intervention.

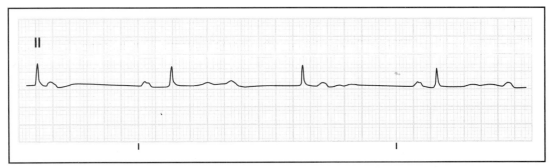

FIGURE 4-8 Your patient's current cardiac rhythm.

From *Arrhythmia Recognition: The Art of Interpretation*, courtesy of Tomas B. Garcia, MD.

Question 3: What medication is indicated first for nonhypovolemic hypotension?

Hypotension that persists despite IV fluid boluses is treated with a dopamine infusion. The dose for dopamine ranges from 2 to 20 mcg/kg/min. It would be most appropriate to begin the infusion at 5 mcg/kg/min and titrate up to 10 mcg/kg/min or until the desired effect is achieved. For severe hypotension, doses of greater than 10 mcg/kg/min may be needed.

Question 4: What other medication could have been used to treat this patient's hypotension?

If dopamine were unsuccessful in raising this patient's blood pressure, an epinephrine infusion would have been the next drug of choice. The correct dose for epinephrine ranges from 2 to 10 mcg/min and should be titrated to the desired effect.

Beyond eACLS Basics: How would your treatment have differed had this been a heart transplant patient?

A transplanted heart does not have an inherent electrical conduction system; it has been denervated and is artificially paced. Atropine would not be effective, as it increases the heart rate by blocking the parasympathetic nervous system via the vagus nerve, which the denervated heart does not have. Initial treatment, therefore, would have been immediate TCP.

eACLS Practice Case 3

A 60-year-old man is found unresponsive and cyanotic. A brief scan of his chest reveals that he is not breathing. You palpate his carotid pulse and determine that it is present. There are no signs of trauma, so you open his airway with the head tilt-chin lift maneuver. You attempt to ventilate him with a pocket face mask; however, his chest does not rise and resistance is met.

Question 1: How will you initially remedy this problem?

Your initial intervention has remedied the problem, and your ventilations now produce a bilateral rise of the patient's chest. Your partner prepares additional equipment.

Question 2: How will you continue to treat this patient?

The appropriate treatment is continued. Your assistant informs you that he needs to insert an advanced airway device because the patient's cyanosis is worsening. As he gathers the appropriate equipment, you preoxygenate the patient with 100% oxygen.

Question 3: When should you insert an advanced airway device in an apneic patient?

Your partner has secured the patient's airway with an advanced airway device, and ventilations are continued at the appropriate rate. Auscultation reveals negative epigastric sounds and bilaterally equal lung sounds.

Question 4: What should you do to further confirm proper advanced airway placement?

Correct advanced airway placement has been confirmed with an appropriate additional method, and ventilations with 100% oxygen are continued at a rate of 10 to 12 breaths per minute. The patient's pulse rate, which was initially rapid, has decreased to a normal rate. His skin is now pink.

Question 5: What is the correct ventilatory duration and tidal volume for a patient with an advanced airway in place?

The patient is placed on a mechanical ventilator, and the rate and tidal volume are set accordingly. He is transferred for continued care, where an assessment to determine the cause of his respiratory arrest is performed.

Beyond eACLS Basics

What are the hazards of hyperventilating an apneic patient?

eACLS Practice Case 3 Summary

Question 1: How will you initially remedy this problem?

If initial ventilation attempts fail to produce a chest rise or if you meet resistance, your initial intervention is to reposition the patient's head and reattempt to ventilate. Often, the patient's head was not placed in the appropriate position initially.

Question 2: How will you continue to treat this patient?

This patient is in respiratory arrest with a pulse. You must treat this patient by providing positive-pressure ventilations at a rate of 10 to 12 breaths per minute (1 breath every 5 to 6 seconds) with a bag mask or a pocket mask device that is attached to 100% oxygen.

Question 3: When should you insert an advanced airway device in an apneic patient?

Initial ventilations for an apneic patient should be provided with basic methods; insert an oropharyngeal or nasopharyngeal airway and ventilate the patient with a bag-mask device or a pocket mask device. If, however, the rescuer is unable to ventilate the patient effectively with basic methods, an advanced airway (ie, ET tube, King LT, supraglottic airway [ie, LMA, CobraPLA]) should be inserted. The patient in this case is remaining cyanotic, which indicates ineffective bag-mask ventilation.

Question 4: What should you do to further confirm proper advanced airway placement?

In addition to auscultating the epigastrium and lung fields, quantitative waveform capnography should be used to confirm proper advanced airway placement, as well as to monitor ongoing advanced airway placement.

If the advanced airway is properly placed and ventilations are provided at the proper rate, you should expect to see a normal capnographic waveform and an $ETCO_2$ reading (per LED) between 35 and 45 mm Hg.

If the advanced airway is improperly placed (eg, an ET tube that is in the esophagus), you will not see a capnographic waveform or an LED reading.

Question 5: What is the correct ventilatory duration and tidal volume for a patient with an advanced airway device in place?

Whether you are ventilating an apneic patient with a bag-mask device or through an advanced airway device, you should deliver each breath over a period of 1 second—just enough to produce visible chest rise. The exact tidal volume required to achieve this varies from person to person, but is generally about 500 mL per breath in the adult.

Beyond eACLS Basics: What are the hazards of hyperventilating an apneic patient?

Hyperventilation of the apneic patient has been shown to cause several negative effects. These include increased intrathoracic pressure, which reduces cardiac output by impeding venous return to the right side of the heart, decreased cerebral perfusion pressure secondary to hyperventilation-induced cerebral vasoconstriction, and an "auto-positive-end expiratory pressure (PEEP)" effect, which is caused by inadequate exhalation and leads to air trapping in the lungs.

eACLS Practice Case 4

A 59-year-old male is found unconscious and cyanotic. Your assessment reveals that he is apneic and pulseless. You immediately begin CPR as your partner retrieves the AED. With CPR in progress, your partner applies the AED pads to the patient's bare chest.

Question 1: What must you do before analyzing this patient's cardiac rhythm?

The AED states "shock advised." After delivering one shock, you immediately resume CPR, starting with chest compressions. Your partner quickly gathers additional equipment.

Question 2: What is your next course of action?

After 2 minutes of additional treatment, you reanalyze the patient's cardiac rhythm and receive a "check patient" message. The patient is still pulseless and apneic.

Question 3: Why would the AED give a "check patient" message?

You check the patient as directed and reanalyze his cardiac rhythm. After receiving a "shock advised" message, you ensure that both you and your partner are clear of the patient, deliver the shock, and immediately resume CPR, starting with chest compressions. Following 2 minutes of CPR, you reanalyze the patient's cardiac rhythm and receive a "no shock advised" message.

Question 4: What must you do after receiving a "no shock advised" message?

A carotid pulse has been restored, but the patient remains apneic. Your partner continues providing positive-pressure ventilations at 10 to 12 breaths per minute as you prepare to transfer the patient for advanced life support care.

Question 5: What should you do if this patient rearrests in your presence?

After advanced life support interventions, the patient's condition continues to improve. Within 15 minutes after spontaneous circulation was restored, he has regained spontaneous breathing and is now awake.

Beyond eACLS Basics

How should you place the AED electrodes in patients with an automated implanted cardioverter/defibrillator (AICD)?

eACLS Practice Case 4 Summary

Question 1: What must you do before analyzing this patient's cardiac rhythm?

You must ensure that no one is touching the patient. The AED will not analyze the patient's cardiac rhythm if movement is detected; therefore, all contact with the patient must cease.

Question 2: What is your next course of action?

Following defibrillation, you should *immediately* resume CPR for 2 minutes, starting with chest compressions. During this time, an airway adjunct should be applied, and ventilations should be initiated with a bag-mask or a pocket mask device. Be sure to attach supplemental oxygen to the ventilatory device that you are using. Following 2 minutes of CPR, you should reanalyze the patient's cardiac rhythm.

Question 3: Why would the AED give a "check patient" message?

A "check patient" message indicates that physical contact with the patient has occurred during the analysis phase or one of the AED electrodes has detached from the patient's chest. You must quickly remedy the problem so that the AED can analyze the patient's cardiac rhythm.

Question 4: What must you do after receiving a "no shock advised" message?

If the AED states "no shock advised," you should immediately resume CPR for 2 minutes and then reassess the patient. If the patient has a carotid pulse, you should assess breathing and continue to treat accordingly. If the patient does not have a carotid pulse, reanalyze the cardiac rhythm again.

Question 5: What should you do if this patient rearrests in your presence?

If the patient rearrests, you should immediately analyze his cardiac rhythm with the AED and deliver another shock if indicated. Following this shock, immediately perform CPR, starting with chest compressions, for 2 minutes. After 2 minutes of CPR, reanalyze the patient's cardiac rhythm and deliver another shock if indicated. Continue CPR for 2 minutes, followed by analysis of the patient's cardiac rhythm (and defibrillation, if indicated) until ALS personnel arrive or the patient starts to move. Never remove the AED from patients who have been resuscitated from cardiac arrest; they remain at high risk for recurrent cardiac arrest.

Beyond eACLS Basics: How should you place the AED electrodes in patients with an automated implanted cardioverter/defibrillator (AICD)?

If the patient has an AICD or implanted pacemaker device, it will be palpable as a hard lump underneath the skin, typically on the patient's upper left chest. Placing the AED electrode directly over the implanted device may reduce the effectiveness of defibrillation. You should place the AED electrode at least 1 inch away from the implanted device.

eACLS Practice Case 5

A 65-year-old woman with a history of hypertension experiences a sudden onset of left-sided weakness, confusion, and slurred speech. Her daughter tells you that this began approximately 30 minutes ago. The pulse oximeter reads 92% on room air; therefore, the patient is placed on oxygen with a nasal cannula.

Question 1: Why is it important to establish the onset of symptoms in this patient?

The patient's blood pressure is 148/90 mm Hg. The pulse rate is 70 beats per minute and irregular, and respirations are 16 breaths per minute and unlabored. Further assessment of the patient reveals marked weakness to the left side of her body and a left-sided facial droop.

Question 2: What three physical signs may help you identify this patient's problem?

The patient is placed on a cardiac monitor, which reveals atrial fibrillation at a rate of 70 beats per minute. There are no signs of myocardial ischemia or injury on her 12-lead tracing.

Question 3: How could atrial fibrillation contribute to this patient's problem?

The patient remains conscious, although confused. An IV line of normal saline is established and set at a KVO rate. Blood is also drawn for chemistry and coagulation analysis.

Question 4: What blood test can quickly exclude a possible cause of this patient's problem?

The patient's condition remains unchanged. You notify receiving personnel of your impending arrival and apprise them of the patient's presentation, assessment findings, your interventions, and her present condition.

Question 5: What is the timeframe for drug therapy after this patient reaches the hospital door?

The physician sees the patient within 10 minutes of arrival in the emergency department. Radiographic confirmation of her condition is obtained, and after the appropriate drug therapy is initiated, her neurologic deficits improve.

Beyond eACLS Basics

Why is D_5W contraindicated for this patient?

eACLS Practice Case 5 Summary

Question 1: Why is it important to establish the onset of symptoms in this patient?

This patient is displaying signs of an acute ischemic stroke. Establishing when the symptoms first began will determine (among other criteria) her eligibility for fibrinolytic therapy.

Question 2: What three physical signs may help you identify this patient's problem?

The Cincinnati Prehospital Stroke Scale identifies a potential stroke patient by assessing three physical findings: facial droop, motor arm drift, and speech difficulties. According to the American Heart Association, if a patient has an abnormality in any one of these three physical findings (as a new event), there is a 72% probability that he or she is suffering from an acute ischemic stroke. If all three signs are abnormal, there is a greater than 85% probability of an acute ischemic stroke. Paramedics can use the Cincinnati Prehospital Stroke Scale to determine the likelihood of a stroke. Hospital personnel such as nurses and physicians commonly use the National Institutes of Health (NIH) Stroke Scale, which includes parameters such as a patient's level of consciousness, awareness, and muscle strength.

Question 3: How could atrial fibrillation contribute to this patient's problem?

Atrial fibrillation can result in microemboli formation in the atria, which could travel to the brain and block a cerebral artery. Because of decreased atrial contractile force that accompanies atrial fibrillation, blood can stagnate in the atria, causing small clots.

Question 4: What blood test can quickly exclude a possible cause of this patient's problem?

Assessment of the patient's blood glucose level can exclude hypoglycemia, which can mimic certain signs of a stroke, such as confusion and slurred speech. You should routinely assess the blood glucose level of any patient with an altered mental status and administer dextrose if it is less than 70 mg/dL with signs and symptoms.

Question 5: What is the timeframe for drug therapy after this patient reaches the hospital door?

The National Institute of Neurologic Disorders and Stroke (NINDS) recommends that the time target for fibrinolytic therapy initiation is within 60 minutes after the patient reaches the hospital door.

Beyond eACLS Basics: Why is D₅W contraindicated for this patient?

Hypotonic solutions such as D_5W are contraindicated in patients suspected of having a stroke because they can cause an abrupt fall in serum sodium levels and osmolality (concentration), as well as a shift of intravascular fluid that can result in cerebral edema and increased intracranial pressure.

eACLS Practice Case 6

A 48-year-old man presents with a feeling of "fluttering in his chest" that began 1 hour previous. He is conscious and alert and denies shortness of breath or chest discomfort. His blood pressure is 130/70 mm Hg. His pulse rate is 170 beats per minute and strong, and respirations are 16 breaths per minute and unlabored. The pulse oximeter reads 93% on room air.

Question 1: What should your first intervention be for this patient?

The ECG leads are attached to the patient, and his cardiac rhythm is assessed (FIGURE 4-9). As your assistant is initiating an IV line of normal saline, you prepare to perform a therapeutic intervention.

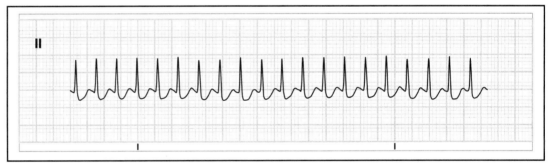

FIGURE 4-9 Your patient's cardiac rhythm.

From *Arrhythmia Recognition: The Art of Interpretation*, courtesy of Tomas B. Garcia, MD.

Question 2: What intervention is used initially to slow this patient's heart rate?

After your initial intervention, the patient's condition and cardiac rhythm remain unchanged. Your assistant informs you that a patent IV line is now running. You open the medication box in preparation for your next intervention.

Question 3: What is the next treatment intervention for this patient?

The patient tells you that he has become short of breath. His skin is pale and diaphoretic, his pulse is weak, and his oxygen saturation is now 89%. You reassess his blood pressure and note that it is 84/50 mm Hg. After providing a higher concentration of oxygen, you prepare for further treatment. Your assistant hands you a syringe containing midazolam.

Question 4: What treatment intervention is indicated for this patient now?

After your next treatment intervention, you note a change in the patient's cardiac rhythm (FIGURE 4-10). His blood pressure is now 128/68 mm Hg. His heart rate is 76 beats per minute and is strong and regular, and his respirations are unlabored. He is no longer short of breath, and the pulse oximeter reads 98%.

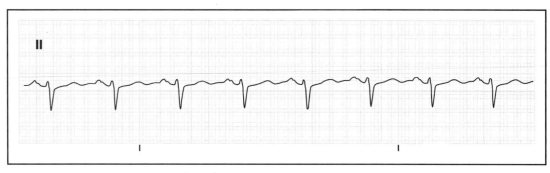

FIGURE 4-10 Your patient's current cardiac rhythm.

From *Arrhythmia Recognition: The Art of Interpretation*, courtesy of Tomas B. Garcia, MD.

Question 5: How will you complete your treatment of this patient?

Once at the emergency department, a 12-lead ECG is obtained, which reveals a normal sinus rhythm, and blood is drawn for electrolyte analysis. The patient's condition remains stable, and he will be on telemetry under observation until the evaluation is complete.

Beyond eACLS Basics

Why would multifocal atrial tachycardia NOT respond to synchronized cardioversion?

eACLS Practice Case 6 Summary

Question 1: What should your first intervention be for this patient?

Your patient's oxygen saturation is 93%; therefore, supplemental oxygen via nasal cannula (2 to 4 L/min) would be appropriate. If the patient's oxygen saturation continues to drop or if he develops respiratory distress, a higher concentration of oxygen should be administered.

Question 2: What intervention is used initially to slow this patient's heart rate?

The patient is displaying a narrow complex tachycardia at 170 to 180 beats per minute. Because he is not exhibiting serious signs and symptoms linked to the tachycardia, he is stable. The initial intervention to slow the patient's heart rate is to perform vagal maneuvers. Techniques such as coughing, immersing the patient's face in ice-cold water (diving reflex), breath-holding, and bearing down (Valsalva maneuver) can be used safely.

Question 3: What is the next treatment intervention for this patient?

Because the patient remains stable and has not responded to vagal maneuvers, the next treatment of choice is to administer adenosine 6 mg via a rapid (over 1 to 3 seconds) IV push, followed by a 20-mL normal saline flush. Elevate the patient's arm to facilitate rapid delivery of the drug. If 6 mg of adenosine is unsuccessful, you may administer 12 mg after 2 minutes, if needed.

Question 4: What treatment intervention is indicated for this patient now?

Your patient has developed serious signs and symptoms as the result of his narrow complex tachycardia and is therefore unstable. Treatment must now include synchronized cardioversion, starting with 50 to 100 biphasic joules. If your initial cardioversion attempt is unsuccessful, increase the energy setting in a stepwise fashion. Midazolam is used to sedate the patient before cardioversion.

Question 5: How will you complete your treatment of this patient?

You have successfully converted this patient's narrow complex tachycardia with the appropriate intervention. He is presently in a normal sinus rhythm at a rate of approximately 80 beats per minute. It would now be appropriate to transport/transfer him for further care.

Beyond eACLS Basics: Why would multifocal atrial tachycardia NOT respond to synchronized cardioversion?

Multifocal atrial tachycardia and junctional tachycardia are both caused by an automatic or "irritable" focus and will not respond to synchronized cardioversion. Rhythms such as paroxysmal supraventricular tachycardia are caused by a reentry circuit within the AV junction and will generally respond well to cardioversion. Determining the underlying rhythm when a stable patient presents with a narrow complex tachycardia will enable you to select the appropriate treatment.

eACLS Practice Case 7

A 58-year-old woman complains of a sudden onset of substernal chest discomfort, nausea, and diaphoresis that began 2 hours ago. She tells you that she has coronary artery disease and has taken three nitroglycerin tablets without relief. Oxygen is placed at 4 L/min via a nasal cannula, and your assistant prepares to start an IV line of normal saline.

Question 1: Other than oxygen, what treatment can you provide to this patient without IV access?

The IV line is patent and running at a KVO rate. The patient's blood pressure is 148/90 mm Hg. Her pulse rate is 120 beats per minute and regular, and her respirations are 22 breaths per minute and unlabored. Your assistant attaches the ECG electrodes to the patient's chest and obtains a lead II ECG strip (FIGURE 4-11). You prepare for your next intervention.

Question 2: What additional treatment may help to reduce this patient's chest discomfort?

After your next treatment intervention, the patient tells you that her chest discomfort has improved somewhat. A 12-lead ECG tracing shows 3-mm ST-segment elevation in leads II, III, and aVF. A right-sided 12-lead ECG tracing shows no ST-segment elevation in lead V_4R. You ask the patient whether she has any known bleeding disorders or a stroke or recent surgeries.

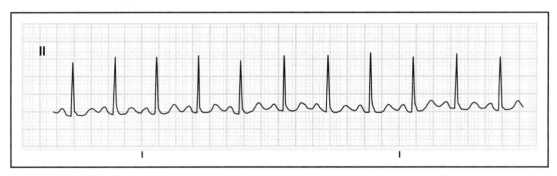

FIGURE 4-11 Your patient's cardiac rhythm.

From *Arrhythmia Recognition: The Art of Interpretation*, courtesy of Tomas B. Garcia, MD.

Question 3: Why are you asking the patient those specific questions?

The patient denies a history of stroke, recent surgeries, or any bleeding disorders. She tells you that her chest discomfort is still present and is beginning to radiate to her jaw. You repeat her blood pressure, which is 130/70 mm Hg.

Question 4: Is further treatment required for this patient?

Reassessment of the patient reveals a blood pressure of 110/80 mm Hg, a pulse rate of 90 beats per minute and regular, and respirations of 18 breaths per minute and unlabored. She is still complaining of slight chest discomfort. You transfer/transport her to the emergency department for definitive care of her condition.

Question 5: What additional tests should you expect the emergency department physician to order?

After additional assessment and laboratory work, a definitive diagnosis of the patient's condition is quickly made in the emergency department, and within 30 minutes of her reaching the emergency department, the appropriate pharmacologic therapy is initiated. Within 20 minutes after this therapy is initiated, she is pain free.

Beyond eACLS Basics
How do fibrinolytic agents work to dissolve a thrombus?

eACLS Practice Case 7 Summary
Question 1: Other than oxygen, what treatment can you provide to this patient without IV access?
Aspirin (162 to 324 mg [non-enteric coated]) should be given to patients with signs of an ACS as soon as possible. Aspirin has clearly demonstrated decreased mortality and morbidity from ACS and should not be delayed for the purpose of starting an IV line.

Question 2: What additional treatment may help to reduce this patient's chest discomfort?
Before ordering morphine or nitroglycerin, review the contraindications and risks to decide if the benefit outweighs these. If three nitroglycerin tablets (or sprays) fail to relieve the patient's chest discomfort completely, you should administer 2 to 4 mg of morphine sulfate via a slow (over 1 to 5 minutes) IV push. You may repeat morphine at 5- to 30-minute intervals. Because morphine is a narcotic analgesic, you must monitor the patient for signs of central nervous system depression (ie, decreased respirations, hypotension) and must be prepared to administer naloxone, a narcotic antagonist.

Question 3: Why are you asking the patient these specific questions?
These specific questions (among others) are asked to determine her eligibility for fibrinolytic therapy, which must be initiated within 12 hours after the onset of symptoms. She has already met the inclusion criteria for fibrinolytic therapy, which is ST-segment elevation that is greater than or equal to 1 mm in two or more contiguous leads, signs of ACS, and the onset of symptoms within the last 12 hours and PCI is not available within 90 minutes of first medical contact.

Question 4: Is further treatment required for this patient?
Because the patient's blood pressure is stable and she is still complaining of chest discomfort, you should administer another dose of morphine (2 to 4 mg). Pain relief is an important aspect in the management of a patient with an ACS, as pain increases anxiety, thus increasing myocardial oxygen demand and consumption. This effect could extend (enlarge) her myocardial infarction and potentially cause cardiogenic shock or cardiac arrest.

Question 5: What additional tests should you expect the emergency department physician to order?
The impressive 12-lead findings clearly indicate inferior wall myocardial infarction; however, the physician will also obtain a chest x-ray and blood samples to analyze her cardiac serum markers, blood chemistry, and coagulation times. Further questions will also be asked to confirm her candidacy for fibrinolytic therapy.

Beyond eACLS Basics: How do fibrinolytic agents work to dissolve a thrombus?
Fibrinolytic agents such as tissue plasminogen activator and streptokinase convert free plasminogen to the proteolytic enzyme plasmin. Plasmin in turn degrades the fibrin and fibrinogen matrix of the thrombus, thereby producing lysis (destruction) of the thrombus, hence the term "fibrinolysis."

eACLS Practice Case 8
A 49-year-old male suddenly collapses shortly after complaining of chest discomfort. The patient's wife says that he has had two previous heart attacks, and that he collapsed about 5 minutes prior to your arrival. Your assessment reveals that he is pulseless and apneic. Your assistant begins CPR while you apply the defibrillator pads and assess his cardiac rhythm (FIGURE 4-12).

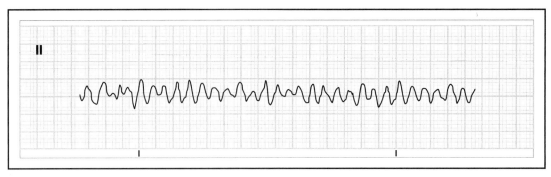

FIGURE 4-12 Your patient's cardiac rhythm.
From *Arrhythmia Recognition: The Art of Interpretation*, courtesy of Tomas B. Garcia, MD.

Question 1: What immediate intervention is indicated for this patient?

Following your intervention, you immediately resume CPR. During this time, two assistants arrive to help you and your partner. An IV line of normal saline is established. Following 2 minutes of CPR, you reassess the patient and determine that his condition is unchanged. You repeat your previous intervention and immediately resume CPR.

Question 2: What pharmacologic intervention(s) should be given first?

The first medication is administered and circulated with effective CPR. Following 2 minutes of CPR, you reassess the patient and determine that his condition remains unchanged. The patient has also been successfully intubated.

Question 3: What intervention is indicated next for this patient?

Following your next intervention, your two assistants immediately resume CPR. Your partner hands you the next medication indicated for this patient's condition.

Question 4: What pharmacologic intervention should be given next?

You administer the next pharmacologic agent for the patient while CPR is ongoing. After 2 minutes, you perform an electrical intervention and immediately resume CPR. After 2 minutes of CPR, you reassess the patient and note that his cardiac rhythm has changed (FIGURE 4-13). The patient now has a palpable carotid pulse.

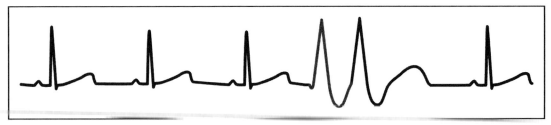

FIGURE 4-13 Your patient's current cardiac rhythm.
From *Arrhythmia Recognition: The Art of Interpretation*, courtesy of Tomas B. Garcia, MD.

The patient remains apneic, so positive pressure ventilations are continued. The patient's blood pressure is 100/70 mm Hg, and his heart rate is 76 beats per minute and irregular. You prepare an intervention to prevent a recurrence of his presenting dysrhythmia.

Question 5: What intervention will prevent a recurrence of this patient's presenting dysrhythmia?

The appropriate intervention has been performed. The patient's cardiac rhythm now shows a normal sinus rhythm at a rate of 70 beats per minute and no ectopy. His blood pressure remains stable, and the pulse oximetry reads 99% (intubated and receiving ventilations). You transport/transfer him for further stabilization of his condition.

Beyond eACLS Basics

What might this patient's presenting dysrhythmia have looked like if he had been hypomagnesemic?

eACLS Practice Case 8 Summary

Question 1: What immediate intervention is indicated for this patient?

This patient requires immediate defibrillation with 360 joules monophasic (or biphasic equivalent). He is in V-fib, the most important treatment for which is prompt defibrillation. Ensure that no one is touching the patient before defibrillating. Following defibrillation, you should immediately resume CPR and reassess the patient's condition in 2 minutes.

Question 2: What pharmacologic intervention(s) should be given first?

One of two possible medications can be given to this patient as the initial pharmacologic intervention. Epinephrine 1 mg 1:10,000 via rapid IV push can be given every 3 to 5 minutes. Vasopressin, in a one-time dose of 40 units, can be used to replace the first or second dose of epinephrine.

Question 3: What intervention is indicated next for this patient?

Because it has been 2 minutes since your last defibrillation attempt and the patient's condition has not changed, you must repeat defibrillation with 360 joules (or biphasic equivalent) and then immediately resume CPR for 2 minutes. After 2 minutes of CPR, reassess the patient and defibrillate again if needed.

Question 4: What pharmacologic intervention should be given next?

For refractory V-fib or pulseless V-tach, you can administer one of the following antiarrhythmic medications:

- Amiodarone: 300 mg via rapid IV push
  - Repeat in 3–5 minutes at 150 mg via rapid IV push.
- Lidocaine: 1–1.5 mg/kg via rapid IV push
  - Repeat in 5–10 minutes at 0.5–0.75 mg/kg.
  - The maximum dose is 3 mg/kg.

Question 5: What intervention will prevent a recurrence of this patient's presenting dysrhythmia?

An antiarrhythmic maintenance infusion will help prevent a recurrence of V-fib or pulseless V-tach. Begin an infusion of the medication that aided in the conversion of the patient's ventricular dysrhythmia.

- Amiodarone (24-hour maintenance infusion)
  - 360-mg IV over the first 6 hours (1 mg/min) and then 540-mg IV over the remaining 18 hours (0.5 mg/min)
  - The maximum dose is 2.2 g per 24 hours.
- Lidocaine
  - 1–4 mg/min titrated to the desired effect

Preventing recurrent V-fib or pulseless V-tach is a critical aspect of postresuscitation management. If the patient rearrests, the chances of a successful second resuscitation are lower.

Beyond eACLS Basics: What might this patient's presenting dysrhythmia have looked like if he had been hypomagnesemic?

Hypomagnesemia is a very common cause of polymorphic V-tach, which in this patient, would have been treated with defibrillation, but magnesium sulfate 1 to 2 g IV would have been the preferred antiarrhythmic agent. Additionally, prolongation of the Q-T interval can cause torsade de pointes (TdP), a variant of polymorphic V-tach. In these patients, you should avoid the use of medications that prolong the Q-T interval, such as procainamide.

eACLS Practice Case 9

CPR is in progress on a 70-year-old woman who was found unresponsive in her bed. There is no evidence of trauma. You instruct your team to cease CPR temporarily as you assess her cardiac rhythm (FIGURE 4-14).

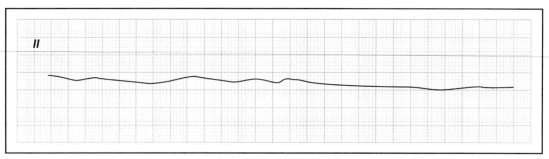

FIGURE 4-14 Your patient's cardiac rhythm.

From *Arrhythmia Recognition: The Art of Interpretation,* courtesy of Tomas B. Garcia, MD.

Question 1: How will you confirm this patient's cardiac rhythm?

The patient's cardiac rhythm has been confirmed. CPR is continued and the ECG leads are attached. An IV line of normal saline has been established and the appropriate airway management is being performed.

Question 2: What pharmacologic agent(s) should be given to this patient first?

The first medication has been administered to the patient, whose condition and cardiac rhythm remain unchanged. As CPR is continued, the rescuer performing ventilations intubates the patient because he was experiencing difficulty ventilating with a bag-mask device. Ventilations are continued at a rate of 8 to 10 breaths per minute.

Question 3: How would you treat acidosis as the cause of this patient's condition?

Measures are taken to treat the hypoxia and acidosis associated with the patient's condition. As other potential causes of her condition are excluded, you prepare for your next intervention.

Question 4: What are some other potentially reversible causes of this patient's cardiac arrest?

CPR continues while you search for other potentially reversible causes of her cardiac arrest. Her blood glucose level reads 90 mg/dL, there is no evidence of hypovolemia or trauma, and her breath sounds are clear and equal bilaterally. You elicit feedback from your team regarding the cessation of resuscitative efforts.

Question 5: What factors should be considered when determining whether resuscitative efforts should cease?

You have exhausted all efforts at resuscitating this patient, and the decision is made to cease further resuscitative efforts. The patient's family is contacted and apprised of the situation. They agree with your decision.

Beyond eACLS Basics

Why is defibrillation not recommended for this patient's cardiac rhythm?

eACLS Practice Case 9 Summary
Question 1: How will you confirm this patient's cardiac rhythm?

When asystole presents on the cardiac monitor, you should assess another lead to ensure that it is not actually fine V-fib. You should also increase the gain sensitivity on the cardiac monitor. If fine V-fib is suspected or confirmed, defibrillate the patient at once.

Question 2: What pharmacologic agent(s) should be given to this patient first?

One of two possible medications can be given to this patient as the initial pharmacologic intervention. Epinephrine 1 mg 1:10,000 via rapid IV push can be given every 3 to 5 minutes. Vasopressin, in a one-time dose of 40 units, can be used to replace the first or second dose of epinephrine.

Question 3: How would you treat acidosis associated with this patient's condition?

Acidosis is present to some degree in all patients with cardiac arrest and worsens as the arrest persists. Initial treatment for acidosis, regardless of the cause, is to ensure adequate oxygenation and ventilation. Measures should be taken, such as confirming correct advanced airway placement and ensuring the delivery of 100% oxygen. If lactic acidosis is confirmed with an arterial blood gas, sodium bicarbonate should be given.

Question 4: What are some other potentially reversible causes of this patient's cardiac arrest?

Any patient in cardiac arrest—regardless of his or her presenting cardiac rhythm—should be assessed for underlying causes that, if detected and corrected early, may facilitate return of spontaneous circulation (ROSC). In addition to hypoxia and acidosis, other potentially reversible causes of cardiac arrest include hypothermia, hypoglycemia, hypo- or hyperkalemia, drug overdose, tension pneumothorax, cardiac tamponade, pulmonary or coronary thrombus, and trauma.

Some of these potentially reversible causes can be ruled out through a physical exam, such as tension pneumothorax, cardiac tamponade, hypothermia, and trauma. Others, such as hypo- or hyperkalemia, should be suspected if the patient's history is suggestive (ie, severe vomiting and/or diarrhea, dialysis patient), but require blood chemistry analysis to rule out definitively.

In addition to treating the patient with CPR, airway management, and appropriate drug therapy, it is critical to *actively assess* for potentially reversible causes that may have caused, or are contributing to, the patient's cardiac arrest.

Question 5: What factors should be considered when determining whether resuscitative efforts should cease?

The decision to terminate resuscitative efforts is one that must not be taken lightly. The following criteria should be used when contemplating termination of resuscitative efforts in a patient with asystole:

- Was high-quality CPR (with minimal interruption) performed throughout the entire arrest?
- If V-fib was present, was it terminated with defibrillation?
- Was an advanced airway placed, confirmed with quantitative waveform capnography, and maintained throughout the arrest?
- Was vascular access established, with all rhythm-appropriate medications administered?
- Were potentially reversible causes of the asystole treated or ruled out?
- Has asystole persisted for more than 10 minutes, after all appropriate therapies have been administered?
- Have family members been apprised of the situation and do they object to cessation of resuscitative efforts?

Beyond eACLS Basics: Why is defibrillation not recommended for this patient's cardiac rhythm?

There are no valid data that suggest that routine defibrillation of asystolic patients yields a better outcome than without defibrillation. In fact, defibrillating asystolic patients can be harmful, as it can produce a "stunned" heart and profound parasympathetic discharge, thus eliminating any possibility of restoring spontaneous cardiac electrical activity. Additionally, defibrillating asystolic patients can significantly reduce, if not eliminate, the chances of treating any potentially reversible underlying causes.

eACLS Practice Case 10

You arrive at the site about 5 minutes after a 55-year-old man collapsed. According to the patient's wife, he had been complaining of vomiting, diarrhea, and progressive weakness over the past 2 days. There is no history of trauma. Your primary assessment reveals that he is pale, pulseless, and apneic. CPR is initiated and you assess his cardiac rhythm (FIGURE 4-15).

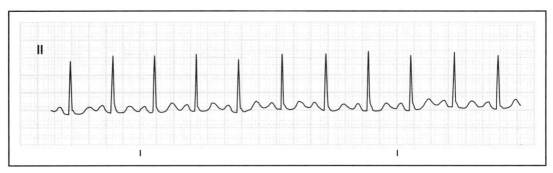

FIGURE 4-15 Your patient's cardiac rhythm.
From *Arrhythmia Recognition: The Art of Interpretation*, courtesy of Tomas B. Garcia, MD.

Question 1: How would you define this patient's condition?

CPR is continued as a patent IV line of normal saline is established, and preparations for ET intubation are made. The patient's wife states that other than the recent illness, her husband is relatively healthy and takes no medications.

Question 2: What pharmacologic agent(s) should be given to this patient first?

The first medication for this patient's condition has been administered and is being circulated with effective CPR. The patient has been intubated, and your assistant reports clear and equal breath sounds and increased ventilatory compliance. Proper tube placement is confirmed with quantitative waveform capnography.

Question 3: Based on his presentation, what do you suspect to be the cause of this patient's condition?

A 500-mL bolus of normal saline is administered, and the patient is reassessed. He remains pulseless and apneic, with no change in his cardiac rhythm. Additional normal saline boluses are given as CPR is continued.

Question 4: Why would you NOT suspect a tension pneumothorax as the cause of this patient's condition?

After additional normal saline boluses, a carotid pulse is now palpable. You assess the patient's airway and continue ventilatory support. The patient's blood pressure is palpated at 70 mm Hg systolic. He is immediately transferred for further stabilization.

Question 5: What is commonly associated with the underlying cause of this patient's problem?

The patient continues to improve, and he is now in a normal sinus rhythm. After further stabilization in the emergency department, he is admitted to the medical intensive care unit and discharged home after a 10-day stay in the hospital.

Beyond eACLS Basics

What are the "obstructive" causes of this patient's condition?

eACLS Practice Case 10 Summary

Question 1: How would you define this patient's condition?

This patient is in pulseless electrical activity (PEA). He has a cardiac rhythm (sinus tachycardia) on the monitor, but does not have a detectable pulse.

Question 2: What pharmacologic agent(s) should be given to this patient first?

One of two possible medications can be given to this patient as the initial pharmacologic intervention. Epinephrine 1 mg 1:10,000 via rapid IV push can be given every 3 to 5 minutes. Vasopressin, in a one-time dose of 40 units, can be used to replace the first or second dose of epinephrine.

Question 3: Based on his presentation, what do you suspect to be the cause of this patient's condition?

With a 2-day history of severe vomiting and diarrhea, which has no doubt led to profound dehydration, you should be extremely suspicious for hypovolemia as the primary cause of his PEA. The narrow complex tachycardia and his pallor are also indicators of hypovolemic PEA. Hypovolemia is perhaps the most easily reversible cause of PEA, and thus, aggressive fluid resuscitation is needed with frequent reassessments of the patient. It is acceptable to give an "empiric medical bolus" of 500 mL of normal saline, even without specific evidence of hypovolemia.

Question 4: Why would you NOT suspect a tension pneumothorax as the cause of this patient's condition?

The patient's breath sounds are clear and equal bilaterally, and your assistant is not having difficulty ventilating the patient. A tension pneumothorax, although commonly associated with a narrow complex tachycardia, typically presents with a slow ventricular rate because of the accompanying hypoxia. This patient's history does not suggest the possibility of a tension pneumothorax.

Question 5: What is commonly associated with the underlying cause of this patient's problem?

Electrolyte depletion is frequently associated with severe dehydration. As fluid is lost from the body, so are electrolytes (ie, sodium, potassium). Hypokalemia should be suspected when the T waves are flattened and prominent U waves exist. Although typically associated with wide QRS complexes, this patient is no doubt somewhat hypokalemic and hyponatremic, both of which need to be treated.

Beyond eACLS Basics: What are the "obstructive" causes of this patient's condition?

The obstructive causes of PEA are tension pneumothorax, pericardial tamponade, coronary thrombosis, and pulmonary embolism. The term "obstructive" means that blood flow is physically restricted (obstructed). A tension pneumothorax obstructs blood flow to the body because of myocardial and great vessel compression. A pericardial tamponade obstructs blood flow to the body as well because of myocardial compression caused by excessive blood or fluid in the pericardial sac. A pulmonary embolism obstructs blood flow to the lungs because of a blocked pulmonary artery. A coronary thrombosis causes obstruction of coronary flow to the heart muscle and results in heart damage (ie, MI).

eACLS Practice Test

Introduction

This section contains a 40-question practice test that is designed to help you prepare for the final eACLS examination and to assist you in identifying potential weak areas. The questions in this practice test are similar to what you will encounter on the final eACLS examination. At the end of the practice test, you will find the correct answers and rationales.

To obtain a reliable assessment of your baseline knowledge of the material, it is recommended that you complete the practice test in its entirety and then refer to the correct answers and rationales.

1. Immediate transcutaneous cardiac pacing (TCP) is indicated for which of the following conditions?
   a. Asymptomatic bradycardia
   b. Pulseless electrical activity
   c. Unstable ventricular tachycardia
   d. Complete heart block with hypotension

2. Which of the following medications is indicated for a hemodynamically stable patient with a wide complex tachycardia?
   a. Atropine
   b. Amiodarone
   c. Morphine
   d. Nitroglycerin

3. A middle-aged woman presents with a narrow complex bradycardia at a rate of 45 beats per minute. Her blood pressure is 80/40 mm Hg, her oxygen saturation is 89%, and she is complaining of chest discomfort. Your FIRST action should be to:
   a. start an IV and give atropine.
   b. obtain a 12-lead ECG tracing.
   c. give supplemental oxygen.
   d. begin a dopamine infusion.

4. The Cincinnati Prehospital Stroke Scale consists of which of the following three assessment tests?
   a. Facial droop, arm drift, abnormal speech
   b. Arm drift, mental status, abnormal speech
   c. Mental status, facial droop, blood pressure
   d. Arm drift, facial droop, mental status

5. Streptokinase falls under which of the following drug classifications?
   a. Antiarrhythmic
   b. Parasympatholytic
   c. Fibrinolytic
   d. Narcotic

6. Your patient presents with the following cardiac rhythm:

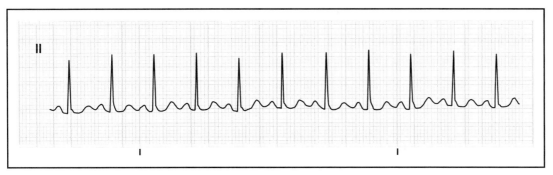

FIGURE A-1 Patient ECG strip.
From Arrhythmia Recognition: The Art of Interpretation, courtesy of Tomas B. Garcia, MD.

Treatment for this cardiac rhythm should focus primarily on:
   a. synchronized cardioversion.
   b. treatment of the cause of the rhythm.
   c. administration of a normal saline bolus.
   d. administration of a sedative drug.

7. A 50-year-old male with a history of coronary artery disease presents with acute chest discomfort, nausea, and shortness of breath. Which of the following treatment modalities are appropriate for this patient?
   a. Obtain a 12-lead ECG tracing.
   b. Obtain intravenous access.
   c. Provide aspirin and nitroglycerin (if blood pressure warrants).
   d. All of the above.

8. Which of the following medications will prolong the Q-T interval?
   a. Epinephrine
   b. Lidocaine
   c. Magnesium
   d. Procainamide

9. An older female patient is in cardiac arrest and presents with the following cardiac rhythm:

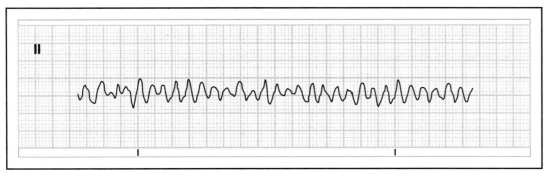

FIGURE A-2 Patient ECG strip.
From Arrhythmia Recognition: The Art of Interpretation, courtesy of Tomas B. Garcia, MD.

Your FIRST action in treating the above cardiac rhythm should be to:
a. start an IV and administer epinephrine.
b. defibrillate one time and initiate CPR.
c. perform immediate synchronized cardioversion.
d. perform high-quality CPR for at least 5 minutes.

10. Which of the following statements regarding vasopressin is correct?
a. Vasopressin is given to all adult cardiac arrest patients in a dose of 20 units every 3–5 minutes.
b. Vasopressin is used to replace the first or second dose of epinephrine for adult patients in cardiac arrest.
c. Vasopressin is the preferred initial drug to administer to adult patients with asystole or PEA.
d. Vasopressin should not be administered to adult patients with unwitnessed cardiac arrest.

11. The recommended "door to drug" time for a patient with a suspected acute ischemic stroke is:
a. 10 minutes.
b. 25 minutes.
c. 45 minutes.
d. 60 minutes.

12. Normal saline fluid boluses have failed to increase the blood pressure in a patient with cardiogenic hypotension. Your next intervention should be:
a. atropine.
b. epinephrine.
c. dopamine.
d. procainamide.

13. Which of the following questions is pertinent when determining whether resuscitative efforts of a patient with asystole should cease?
a. Had the patient experienced cardiac arrest in the past?
b. Is the patient between the ages of 35 and 55 years?
c. Has the family selected and notified the funeral home?
d. Was adequate BLS performed throughout the arrest?

14. Which of the following pulseless rhythms is classified and treated as PEA?
a. Idioventricular rhythm
b. Ventricular tachycardia
c. Torsade de pointes
d. Fine ventricular fibrillation

15. Your initial goal in assessing a patient with a narrow complex tachycardia at a rate of 170 beats per minute should be to:
a. identify the presence of serious signs and symptoms.
b. determine what medications the patient is taking.
c. obtain a complete patient medical history.
d. determine whether the patient has any medication allergies.

16. Which of the following drugs is used *specifically* to increase a patient's heart rate?
a. Epinephrine
b. Atropine
c. Dopamine
d. Amiodarone

17. You have just performed synchronized cardioversion with 100 joules on an unstable patient with a wide complex tachycardia. You reassess him and note that his condition is unchanged. You should next:
a. administer 150 mg of amiodarone.
b. attempt transcutaneous cardiac pacing.

    c. repeat the cardioversion with 200 joules.

    d. begin an infusion of an antiarrhythmic drug.

18. Which of the following is considered to be a serious sign or symptom of cardiac compromise?

    a. Headache

    b. Generalized weakness

    c. Lightheadedness

    d. Altered mental status

19. A cardiac rhythm in which the appearances of the QRS complexes differ in shape and amplitude is said to be:

    a. monomorphic.

    b. polymorphic.

    c. supraventricular.

    d. idioventricular.

20. Midazolam is a medication that is commonly used for what purpose?

    a. As an antiarrhythmic

    b. Decreasing rapid heart rates

    c. Increasing slow heart rates

    d. Sedation before cardioversion

21. Which of the following statements regarding narrow complex tachycardias is correct?

    a. They typically originate in a location within the ventricles.

    b. They are rarely associated with serious signs and symptoms.

    c. They generally do not require cardioversion if the rate is less than 150.

    d. They are always treated initially with adenosine, even if unstable.

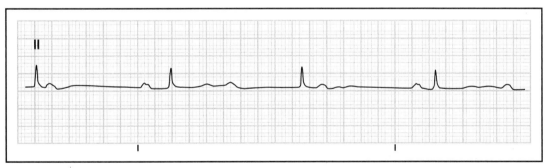

FIGURE A-3 Patient ECG strip.
From Arrhythmia Recognition: The Art of Interpretation, courtesy of Tomas B. Garcia, MD.

22. You should interpret the following cardiac rhythm as:

    a. a third-degree AV block.

    b. sinus bradycardia.

    c. a first-degree AV block.

    d. idioventricular.

23. Which of the following is an example of a "relative" bradycardia?

    a. A heart rate of 65 beats per minute and blood pressure of 110/70 mm Hg

    b. A heart rate of 70 beats per minute and blood pressure of 80/40 mm Hg

    c. A heart rate of 40 beats per minute and blood pressure of 70/50 mm Hg

    d. A heart rate of 50 beats per minute and blood pressure of 120/70 mm Hg

24. You have just defibrillated a patient in V-fib. You look at the cardiac monitor and see what appears to be ventricular tachycardia. You should next:

    a. repeat the defibrillation.

    b. start an IV and give amiodarone.

    c. perform immediate cardioversion.

    d. perform CPR and reassess in 2 minutes.

25. The maximum adult dose for lidocaine is:
   a. 1 mg/kg.
   b. 2 mg/kg.
   c. 3 mg/kg.
   d. 4 mg/kg.

26. Diltiazem would be indicated for which of the following patients?
   a. A 60-year-old male with rapid atrial fibrillation
   b. A 49-year-old female with ventricular fibrillation
   c. A 52-year-old male with sinus bradycardia
   d. A 72-year-old female with a third-degree heart block

27. A 40-year-old male with a narrow complex tachycardia at 170 beats per minute has a stable blood pressure. You should give oxygen, start an IV line, and administer:
   a. cardioversion.
   b. adenosine.
   c. lidocaine.
   d. atropine.

28. Which of the following medications is MOST appropriate to administer to a patient with torsade de pointes?
   a. Procainamide
   b. Amiodarone
   c. Magnesium
   d. Lidocaine

29. All patients with a cardiovascular emergency should receive oxygen if hypoxemic, IV therapy, and:
   a. sublingual nitroglycerin.
   b. cardiac bypass surgery.
   c. cardiac monitoring.
   d. early defibrillation.

30. The correct energy setting for defibrillation for an adult patient is:
   a. 75 joules biphasic or 100 joules monophasic.
   b. 100 joules biphasic or 200 joules monophasic.
   c. 150 joules biphasic or 300 joules monophasic.
   d. 200 or greater joules biphasic or 360 joules monophasic.

31. An older male is found to be unresponsive. You should FIRST:
   a. open his airway.
   b. assess for breathing.
   c. assess his cardiac rhythm.
   d. provide ventilatory support.

32. A 56-year-old male is pulseless and apneic and presents with the following cardiac rhythm:

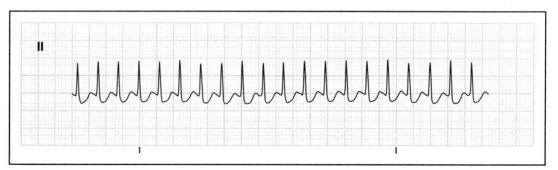

FIGURE A-4 Patient ECG strip.
From Arrhythmia Recognition: The Art of Interpretation, courtesy of Tomas B. Garcia, MD.

Treatment for this patient is likely to include which of the following?
  a. Synchronized cardioversion
  b. Adenosine 6-mg rapid IV push
  c. Immediate defibrillation
  d. Normal saline fluid boluses

33. A 60-year-old man complains of severe chest discomfort. He has been given 324 mg of aspirin and he is receiving oxygen. Despite three nitroglycerin treatments, his pain persists. An IV line has been established and his blood pressure is 148/90 mm Hg. Your next intervention should be to:
  a. repeat the aspirin therapy.
  b. administer 2 to 4 mg of morphine.
  c. administer a saline fluid bolus.
  d. begin an infusion of dopamine.

34. Ventricular fibrillation is a cardiac dysrhythmia that is MOST commonly seen:
  a. early in cardiac arrest in public places.
  b. in patients with chest pain.
  c. in patients with a weak pulse.
  d. as a terminal event.

35. A 40-year-old female presents with a headache and the following rhythm:

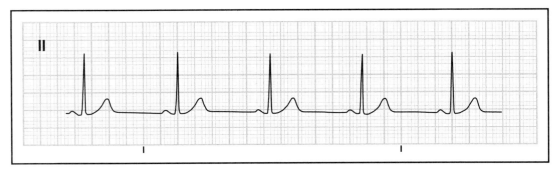

FIGURE A-5 Patient ECG strip.
From Arrhythmia Recognition: The Art of Interpretation, courtesy of Tomas B. Garcia, MD.

Her blood pressure is 118/58 mm Hg, and her pulse is strong. She is conscious and alert and denies chest pain or shortness of breath. Treatment for her should include:
  a. 0.5 mg of atropine sulfate.
  b. transcutaneous cardiac pacing.
  c. continuous cardiac monitoring.
  d. an infusion of epinephrine.

36. Which of the following general statements regarding patient assessment is correct?
  a. Treatment for a patient should be based solely on his or her blood pressure.
  b. A careful and systematic assessment determines the need for treatment.
  c. The absence of chest pain or discomfort means the patient is stable.
  d. If a patient is conscious, he or she is breathing adequately.

37. Fibrinolytic therapy should be administered within how many hours after the onset of stroke symptoms?
  a. 4.5
  b. 6
  c. 9
  d. 12

38. A common cause of conditions such as asystole and PEA is:
  a. hyperthermia.
  b. lactic acidosis.
  c. hypothyroidism.
  d. hyperglycemia.

39. A 31-year-old male is in cardiac arrest. The cardiac rhythm shows a sinus bradycardia at 40 beats per minute. Assessment reveals absent breath sounds on the right side and jugular venous distention. Treatment for this patient's condition includes:
  a. delivering a 1,000-mL normal saline bolus.
  b. giving higher than usual doses of epinephrine.
  c. performing a needle chest decompression.
  d. performing a needle pericardiocentesis.

40. Which of the following medications would increase myocardial oxygen consumption and demand?
  a. Oxygen
  b. Atropine
  c. Diltiazem
  d. Adenosine

Answers and Rationales

1. D. TCP should be initiated as soon as possible for patients with symptomatic bradycardia, especially when accompanied by second-degree type II or third-degree (complete) heart block. TCP is not indicated for patients with pulseless electrical activity. Unstable ventricular tachycardia with a pulse is treated with synchronized cardioversion, not TCP. Pulseless V-tach is treated with defibrillation.

2. B. Medications used in the treatment of stable wide complex tachycardias include amiodarone, lidocaine, and procainamide. Atropine is used to treat symptomatic bradycardia. Both morphine and nitroglycerin are used to treat chest pain associated with acute coronary syndrome.

3. C. Because the patient's oxygen saturation is low (89%), the first intervention that should be performed is oxygen therapy. Give a concentration of oxygen that is sufficient to maintain her oxygen saturation at greater than 94%. Next, interventions aimed at increasing the patient's heart rate should be performed (i.e., atropine, TCP, dopamine, etc.). A 12-lead ECG should also be performed as it may give further information regarding the patient's cardiac rhythm.

4. A. The Cincinnati Prehospital Stroke Scale consists of three assessment tests: facial droop, arm drift, and abnormal speech. Abnormality in any one of these three tests (as a new event) suggests a high probability of an acute ischemic stroke. Blood pressure and mental status assessment are not part of the Cincinnati Prehospital Stroke Scale.

5. C. Streptokinase is a fibrinolytic agent used to treat acute coronary syndromes, specifically acute myocardial infarction (AMI). Antiarrhythmic drugs include lidocaine and amiodarone. Atropine is an example of a parasympatholytic drug. Morphine is an example of a narcotic drug.

6. B. Sinus tachycardia is a manifestation of an underlying problem, such as fear, pain, fever, hypoxia, or hypovolemia. A careful and systematic assessment must be performed in order to identify and treat the underlying cause, which may include normal saline boluses or the administration of a sedative drug. Narrow complex tachycardia with a ventricular rate of less than 150 beats per minute typically does not require synchronized cardioversion.

7. D. Patients with signs and symptoms of an acute coronary syndrome should be placed on a 12-lead ECG. An IV should be started, aspirin (162 to 324 mg) provided, and nitroglycerin provided if the blood pressure is adequate.

8. D. Procainamide and amiodarone will both cause prolongation of the Q-T interval, which, on the cardiac monitor, represents the period of time between ventricular depolarization and repolarization. Epinephrine increases systemic vascular resistance and does not affect the Q-T interval. Lidocaine suppresses ventricular irritability with no effect on the Q-T interval. Magnesium is used to treat ventricular dysrhythmias associated with a prolonged Q-T interval (eg, torsade de pointes).

9. B. This patient is in ventricular fibrillation. Your first action should be to defibrillate her one time with 360 monophasic joules (or equivalent biphasic), followed immediately by CPR. CPR is then performed for 2 minutes, not 5 minutes, before reassessing the patient's cardiac rhythm to determine if further shocks are indicated. An IV line and epinephrine are appropriate interventions for this patient, but not before defibrillation and CPR. Synchronized cardioversion is used to treat wide or narrow complex tachycardias in patients who have a pulse, but are unstable.

10. B. Vasopressin can be used to replace the first or second dose of epinephrine for adult patients in cardiac arrest, regardless of the presenting cardiac rhythm. It is given in a one-time dose of 40 units via rapid IV push. There is insufficient evidence to support vasopressin as a superior drug to epinephrine and vice versa.

11. D. The National Institute of Neurologic Disorders and Stroke (NINDS) time targets for the patient with a possible acute ischemic stroke after reaching the hospital door are as follows:
    - Assessment by physician: 10 minutes
    - Availability of neurologic specialist: 15 minutes
    - CT scan (completed): 25 minutes
    - CT scan (formal reading): 45 minutes
    - Door to fibrinolytic therapy initiation: 60 minutes
    - Access to neurosurgical expertise: 2 hours
    - Admission to hospital bed (if receiving fibrinolytics): 4.5 hours

12. C. Dopamine is indicated for hypotension, cardiogenic or otherwise, that is refractory to IV fluid boluses and is titrated to the desired effect. Atropine is used to treat symptomatic bradycardia. Epinephrine is an adjunct to atropine for symptomatic bradycardia. Procainamide is an antiarrhythmic drug that may exacerbate hypotension.

13. D. Factors that should be considered when determining whether resuscitative efforts should cease include the performance of adequate BLS throughout the arrest, the administration of rhythm-appropriate medications, obtaining and maintaining a patent airway and adequate ventilation, termination of V-fib if present, whether or not the patient is older than 18 years, and whether or not the arrest is presumed to have been of a primary cardiac origin. You must ensure that the family is updated on the situation; however, it would not be appropriate to contact a funeral home until the patient is pronounced dead.

14. A. Pulseless electrical activity (PEA) is a condition in which organized electrical activity is present on the cardiac monitor despite the absence of a palpable pulse. Idioventricular rhythms, although slow, are organized and are therefore classified and treated as PEA. Pulseless ventricular tachycardia and ventricular fibrillation are both treated with defibrillation and are not treated as PEA. Torsade de pointes, a variant of polymorphic ventricular tachycardia, is also treated with defibrillation; it is not classified and treated as PEA.

15. A. In order to provide the most appropriate treatment for the patient, your initial goal in assessing a patient with a potentially unstable cardiac rhythm is to determine the presence of serious signs and symptoms linked to his or her cardiac rhythm. Obtaining the patient's medical history, determining what medications the patient is taking, and ascertaining medication allergies are important aspects of assessing all patients.

16. B. Atropine is a parasympatholytic drug that is specifically used to increase the heart rate (positive chronotropy) of a patient with symptomatic bradycardia. Both dopamine and epinephrine possess chronotropic properties but are also used to increase myocardial contractility (positive inotropy). Amiodarone is used to control, among other conditions, rapid heart rates.

17. C. If your initial attempt to cardiovert an unstable patient with either a wide or narrow complex tachycardia is unsuccessful, you should immediately repeat cardioversion

at a high energy setting. Antiarrhythmics (eg, amiodarone, lidocaine, procainamide) would be appropriate if the patient were stable. An antiarrhythmic infusion is used to prevent a recurrent wide complex tachycardia after it has been successful with either an antiarrhythmic bolus or cardioversion.

18. D. Serious signs and symptoms of cardiac compromise include chest pain/discomfort, shortness of breath, pulmonary edema, altered mental status, and hypotension. Headache, generalized weakness, and lightheadedness are nonspecific symptoms; they are not considered to be serious signs or symptoms of cardiac compromise.

19. B. A polymorphic rhythm (ie, polymorphic V-tach) has QRS complexes that differ in shape and amplitude (size). A monomorphic rhythm has QRS complexes that are all of the same shape and amplitude. A supraventricular rhythm indicates a cardiac rhythm that originates above (supra) the ventricles and typically has narrow QRS complexes. An idioventricular rhythm originates in the ventricles and is characterized by wide QRS complexes and a slow ventricular rate.

20. D. Midazolam (Versed) is a benzodiazepine drug that is used to induce sedation in patients before performing synchronized cardioversion. Examples of antiarrhythmic drugs include lidocaine and amiodarone. Drugs used to decrease rapid heart rates include adenosine and amiodarone. Drugs used to increase the heart rate include atropine and epinephrine.

21. C. Narrow complex tachycardias with rates of less than 150 beats per minute generally do not require immediate synchronized cardioversion because they are less commonly associated with serious signs and symptoms. A narrow complex tachycardia indicates a supraventricular origin, not ventricular. Narrow complex tachycardias (rates of more than 150 beats per minute) are commonly associated with serious signs and symptoms. Adenosine is used to treat a narrow complex tachycardia in stable patients.

22. A. A third-degree AV block is characterized by QRS complexes and P waves that are completely dissociated from each other and QRS complex widths of greater than 0.12 seconds. Sinus bradycardia has all the components of a normal sinus rhythm; however, the ventricular rate is less than 60 beats per minute. First-degree AV block also has all of the components of a normal sinus rhythm; however, the P-R interval is greater than 0.20 seconds. An idioventricular rhythm is characterized by wide, bizarre QRS complexes, absent P waves, and a slow ventricular rate.

23. B. Relative bradycardia is defined as a heart rate that is slower than one would expect relative to the patient's condition, usually his or her blood pressure. Absolute bradycardia is defined as a heart rate of less than 60 beats per minute. A heart rate of 70 beats per minute is slower than one would expect to see with a patient whose blood pressure is 80/40 mm Hg.

24. D. Immediately following defibrillation, you should perform CPR and reassess the patient's pulse and cardiac rhythm in 2 minutes. CPR should be immediately resumed for 2 minutes following defibrillation, even if a rhythm change is noted on the cardiac monitor. Synchronized cardioversion is an appropriate treatment for unstable patients with a narrow or wide complex tachycardia who have a pulse.

25. C. The maximum adult dose of lidocaine is 3 mg/kg.

26. A. Diltiazem (Cardizem) is a calcium channel-blocking drug that is used to control the rate of atrial fibrillation and atrial flutter and as an adjunct to adenosine for patients with stable narrow complex tachycardias. Patients with V-fib need prompt defibrillation. Bradycardia, including sinus bradycardia and third-degree heart block, requires pacing and/or atropine.

27. B. Adenosine is given to hemodynamically-stable patients with narrow complex tachycardias in an attempt to slow their heart rate and identify the underlying rhythm. Synchronized cardioversion would be appropriate if the patient's blood pressure was low or other serious signs and symptoms were present. Lidocaine is given to patients with wide complex tachycardias. Atropine is given to patients with bradycardia with serious signs and symptoms.

28. C. Torsade de pointes (TdP), a variant of polymorphic ventricular tachycardia, is associated with a prolonged Q-T interval. Because hypomagnesemia is a common cause of Q-T interval prolongation and TdP, magnesium sulfate is the most appropriate medication to administer. Procainamide prolongs the Q-T interval and may exacerbate TdP, perhaps to the point of V-fib; therefore, it is clearly not indicated. Amiodarone and lidocaine are indicated for polymorphic V-tach with a normal Q-T interval.

29. C. Patients with a cardiovascular emergency should receive oxygen (if hypoxemic), aspirin (unless they are allergic to it), IV therapy, and cardiac monitoring. Cardiac dysrhythmias are common in patients with cardiovascular emergencies. Further treatment depends on the patient's clinical status. Nitroglycerin is indicated for patients with an acute coronary syndrome and an adequate blood pressure. Cardiovascular bypass surgery is not always indicated for patients with a cardiovascular emergency; percutaneous coronary interventions (PCI), such as the placement of a stent, are far more common. Early defibrillation is a critical therapy for patients with V-fib and pulseless V-tach.

30. D. The correct energy setting for defibrillation is approximately 200 joules biphasic and 360 joules monophasic.

31. B. Assessment of an unresponsive patient begins by assessing for breathing; this is performed by briefly scanning the patient's chest and observing for movement. If the patient is not breathing (or has agonal gasps), you should assess for a carotid pulse. If a pulse is absent, begin CPR. If a pulse is present but the patient is apneic, perform rescue breathing at a rate of 10 to 12 breaths/min (one breath every 5 to 6 seconds).

32. D. This patient has pulseless electrical activity (PEA), a condition in which a regular cardiac rhythm is present despite the absence of a pulse. A common cause of PEA is hypovolemia. Normal saline fluid boluses would be appropriate treatment for this patient. Narrow complex fast cardiac rhythms that accompany PEA are often associated with hypovolemia. Adenosine would be appropriate if this patient had a pulse and was stable. Synchronized cardioversion would be appropriate if he had a pulse but was unstable. Defibrillation is performed on patients with V-fib and pulseless V-tach.

33. B. Morphine 2 to 4 mg via a slow IV push is appropriate if nitroglycerin fails to completely relieve the chest pain or discomfort associated with an ACS. Dopamine is indicated for severe, nonhypovolemic hypotension; this patient is not hypotensive. Saline fluid boluses are not indicated for this patient because his blood pressure is stable.

34. A. Ventricular fibrillation is the most common dysrhythmia seen in early cardiac arrest that occurs in public places and a pulse does not accompany it. In contrast to V-fib, asystole is generally a terminal event with a high mortality rate.

35. C. This patient is not displaying serious signs and symptoms linked to her sinus bradycardia; therefore, she is considered to be stable. Treatment should include continuous cardiac monitoring. Interventions such as atropine, transcutaneous cardiac pacing, and an epinephrine or dopamine infusion would be appropriate if she were unstable.

36. B. In order to provide the most appropriate treatment, you must perform a careful and systematic assessment of your patient, to include assessing airway and breathing, blood pressure, and the presence of serious signs and symptoms. Treatment decisions are not based on one sole parameter (eg, blood pressure and chest pain). Just because a patient is conscious does not indicate that he or she is breathing adequately.

37. A. Fibrinolytic therapy for most stroke patients must be administered within 3 hours after the onset of symptoms. In carefully selected patients, fibrinolytic therapy can be considered within 3 to 4.5 hours after the onset of symptoms. After 4.5 hours, the risk for permanent neurologic damage increases significantly.

38. B. The Hs that represent the most common causes of asystole and PEA include hypovolemia, hypoxia, hydrogen ions (acidosis), and hypokalemia/hyperkalemia. Hyperglycemia, hyperthermia, and hypothyroidism are not common causes of asystole or PEA.

39. C. This patient is in PEA because of a tension pneumothorax, and needs immediate chest decompression. Signs of a tension pneumothorax include unilaterally absent breath sounds, jugular venous distention, and as a later sign, tracheal deviation away from the affected side. A tension pneumothorax obstructs the flow of blood by compressing the myocardium and great vessels. This patient's problem is not hypovolemic in nature. Higher doses of epinephrine would be of no benefit to this patient. A needle pericardiocentesis is indicated for patients with a pericardial tamponade.

40. B. Any medication that increases heart rate or myocardial contractility will increase myocardial oxygen consumption and demand. Such medications include atropine, epinephrine, and dopamine. Oxygen increases the myocardial oxygen supply. Drugs such as diltiazem and adenosine are used to decrease heart rate; therefore, they would cause a decrease in myocardial oxygen consumption and demand.

Note: Page numbers followed by f and t indicate material in figures and tables respectively.